T0226831

Thyroid Cancer: Current Diagnosis, Management, and Prognostication

Editor

ROBERT L. WITT

OTOLARYNGOLOGIC CLINICS OF NORTH AMERICA

www.oto.theclinics.com

August 2014 • Volume 47 • Number 4

ELSEVIER

1600 John F. Kennedy Boulevard • Suite 1800 • Philadelphia, Pennsylvania, 19103-2899

http://www.oto.theclinics.com

OTOLARYNGOLOGIC CLINICS OF NORTH AMERICA Volume 47, Number 4
August 2014 ISSN 0030-6665, ISBN-13: 978-0-323-32021-4

Editor: Joanne Husovski
Developmental Editor: Susan Showalter

Otolaryngologic Clinics of North America (ISSN 0030-6665) is published bimonthly by Elsevier, Inc., 360 Park Avenue South, New York, NY 10010-1710. Months of issue are February, April, June, August, October, and December. Business and Editorial Offices: 1600 John F. Kennedy Blvd., Suite 1800, Philadelphia, PA 19103-2899. Customer Service Office: 6277 Sea Harbor Drive, Orlando, FL 32887-4800. Periodicals postage paid at New York, NY and additional mailing offices. Subscription prices is $365.00 per year (US individuals), $692.00 per year (US institutions), $175.00 per year (US student/resident), $485.00 per year (Canadian individuals), $876.00 per year (Canadian institutions), $540.00 per year (international individuals), $876.00 per year (international institutions), $270.00 per year (international & Canadian student/resident). Foreign air speed delivery is included in all *Clinics*' subscription prices. All prices are subject to change without notice. **POSTMASTER:** Send address changes to *Otolaryngologic Clinics of North America*, Elsevier Health Sciences Division, Subscription Customer Service, 3251 Riverport Lane, Maryland Heights, MO 63043. **Telephone: 1-800-654-2452 (U.S. and Canada); 314-447-8871 (outside U.S. and Canada). Fax: 314-447-8029. E-mail: journalscustomerservice-usa@elsevier.com (for print support); journalsonlinesupport-usa@elsevier.com (for online support).**

Reprints. For copies of 100 or more of articles in this publication, please contact the Commercial Reprints Department, Elsevier Inc., 360 Park Avenue South, New York, NY 10010-1710. Tel.: 212-633-3874; Fax: 212-633-3820; E-mail: reprints@elsevier.com.

Otolaryngologic Clinics of North America is also published in Spanish by McGraw-Hill Interamericana Editores S.A., P.O. Box 5-237, 06500 Mexico D.F., Mexico.

Otolaryngologic Clinics of North America is covered in *MEDLINE/PubMed (Index Medicus), Current Contents/Clinical Medicine, Excerpta Medica, BIOSIS, Science Citation Index,* and *ISI/BIOMED.*

PROGRAM OBJECTIVE

The goal of the *Otolaryngologic Clinics of North America* is to provide information on the latest trends in patient management, the newest advances; and provide a sound basis for choosing treatment options in the field of otolaryngology.

TARGET AUDIENCE

All practicing physicians and healthcare professionals who provide patient care to otolaryngologic patients.

LEARNING OBJECTIVES

Upon completion of this activity, participants will be able to:

1. Recognize clinician performed thyroid ultrasound.
2. Discuss the clinical applications and implications of molecular testing in thyroid cancer.
3. Review surgical diagnosis and techniques related to thyroid cancer.

ACCREDITATION

The Elsevier Office of Continuing Medical Education (EOCME) is accredited by the Accreditation Council for Continuing Medical Education (ACCME) to provide continuing medical education for physicians.

The EOCME designates this enduring material for a maximum of 15 *AMA PRA Category 1 Credit*(s) ™. Physicians should claim only the credit commensurate with the extent of their participation in the activity.

All other health care professionals requesting continuing education credit for this enduring material will be issued a certificate of participation.

DISCLOSURE OF CONFLICTS OF INTEREST

The EOCME assesses conflict of interest with its instructors, faculty, planners, and other individuals who are in a position to control the content of CME activities. All relevant conflicts of interest that are identified are thoroughly vetted by EOCME for fair balance, scientific objectivity, and patient care recommendations. EOCME is committed to providing its learners with CME activities that promote improvements or quality in healthcare and not a specific proprietary business or a commercial interest.

The planning committee, staff, authors and editors listed below have identified no financial relationships or relationships to products or devices they or their spouse/life partner have with commercial interest related to the content of this CME activity:

Jeffrey Bumpous, MD; Miranda D. Celestre, MD; Katrina Chaung, MD; Marc D. Coltrera, MD; Louise Davies, MD, MS, FACS; William S. Duke, MD; David W. Eisele, MD; Robert L. Ferris, MD, PhD, FACS; F. Christopher Holsinger, MD, FACS; Kristen Helm; Brynne Hunter; Joanne Husovski; Sandy Lavery; Jill McNair; Iain J. Nixon, MBChB, FRCS (ORL-HNS), PhD; Lisa A. Orloff, MD; Ozan B. Ozgursoy, MD; Snehal G. Patel, MD; Edmund Pribitkin, MD, FACS; Santha Priya; Gregory Randolph, MD, FACS, FACE; David W. Schoppy, MD, PhD; Ashok R. Shaha, MD; Charalambos Solomides, MD; Gabriel J. Tsao, MD; Ralph P. Tufano, MD, MBA, FACS; Madalina Tuluc, MD; Robert L. Witt, MD, FACS; Linwah Yip, MD.

The planning committee, staff, authors and editors listed below have identified financial relationships or relationships to products or devices they or their spouse/life partner have with commercial interest related to the content of this CME activity:

Richard T. Kloos, MD has stock ownership and employment affiliation with Veracyte, Inc.

Brendan C. Stack, Jr., MD, FACS, FACE is a consultant/advisor for Hollingsworth, LLP and Davies, Humphries, PLC.

David L. Steward, MD has a research grant from Veracyte.

David J. Terris, MD, FACS is on Speakers Bureau for Johnson & Johnson.

UNAPPROVED/OFF-LABEL USE DISCLOSURE

The EOCME requires CME faculty to disclose to the participants:

1. When products or procedures being discussed are off-label, unlabelled, experimental, and/or investigational (not US Food and Drug Administration (FDA) approved); and
2. Any limitations on the information presented, such as data that are preliminary or that represent ongoing research, interim analyses, and/or unsupported opinions. Faculty may discuss information about pharmaceutical agents that is outside of FDA-approved labelling. This information is intended solely for CME and is not intended to promote off-label use of these medications. If you have any questions, contact the medical affairs department of the manufacturer for the most recent prescribing information.

TO ENROLL

To enroll in the *Otolaryngologic Clinics of North America* Continuing Medical Education program, call customer service at 1-800-654-2452 or sign up online at http://www.theclinics.com/home/cme. The CME program is available to subscribers for an additional annual fee of USD 365.

METHOD OF PARTICIPATION

In order to claim credit, participants must complete the following:

1. Complete enrolment as indicated above.
2. Read the activity.
3. Complete the CME Test and Evaluation. Participants must achieve a score of 70% on the test. All CME Tests and Evaluations must be completed online.

CME INQUIRIES/SPECIAL NEEDS

For all CME inquiries or special needs, please contact elsevierCME@elsevier.com.

Contributors

EDITOR

ROBERT L. WITT, MD, FACS
Professor of Otolaryngology–Head & Neck Surgery, Thomas Jefferson University, Philadelphia, Pennsylvania; Adjunct Professor of Biological Sciences, University of Delaware, Newark, Delaware; Director, Head and Neck Multidisciplinary Clinic, Helen F. Graham Cancer Center, Christiana Care, Newark, Delaware

AUTHORS

JEFFREY BUMPOUS, MD
Professor and Chair, Division of Otolaryngology-Head and Neck Surgery, University of Louisville, Louisville, Kentucky

MIRANDA D. CELESTRE, MD
Division of Otolaryngology-Head and Neck Surgery, University of Louisville, Louisville, Kentucky

KATRINA CHAUNG, MD
Fellow Physician, Department of Otolaryngology, Georgia Regents University, Augusta, Georgia

MARC D. COLTRERA, MD
Professor, Department of OTO-HNS, University of Washington; Chief, OTO-HNS Division, VA Puget Sound, Seattle, Washington

LOUISE DAVIES, MD, MS, FACS
Department of Veterans Affairs Medical Center, VA Outcomes Group, White River Junction, Vermont; Section of Otolaryngology, Geisel School of Medicine at Dartmouth, Hanover, New Hampshire; The Dartmouth Institute for Health Policy and Clinical Practice, Lebanon, New Hampshire

WILLIAM S. DUKE, MD
Assistant Professor, Department of Otolaryngology, Georgia Regents University, Augusta, Georgia

DAVID W. EISELE, MD
Andelot Professor of Laryngology and Otology; Director of Otolaryngology-Head and Neck Surgery; Professor of Anesthesiology and Critical Care Medicine; Professor of Oncology; Johns Hopkins Outpatient Center, The Johns Hopkins University School of Medicine, Baltimore, Maryland

ROBERT L. FERRIS, MD, PhD, FACS
Professor of Head and Neck Surgery, Department of Otolaryngology, University of Pittsburgh Cancer Institute, University of Pittsburgh, Pittsburgh, Pennsylvania

F. CHRISTOPHER HOLSINGER, MD, FACS
Chief, Division of Head and Neck Surgery; Professor, Department of Otolaryngology, Stanford University School of Medicine, Stanford, California

RICHARD T. KLOOS, MD
Senior Medical Director (Endocrinology), Department of Medical Affairs, Veracyte, Inc, South San Francisco, California

IAIN J. NIXON, PhD
Head and Neck Service, Department of Surgery, Memorial Sloan Kettering Cancer Center, New York, New York

LISA A. ORLOFF, MD
Director, Division of Head and Neck and Endocrine Surgery; Professor, Department of Otolaryngology–Head and Neck Surgery, Stanford University, Stanford, California

OZAN B. OZGURSOY, MD
Head and Neck Endocrine Surgery Fellow, Department of Otolaryngology-Head and Neck Surgery, Johns Hopkins Outpatient Center, The Johns Hopkins University School of Medicine, Baltimore, Maryland

SNEHAL G. PATEL, MD
Head and Neck Service, Department of Surgery, Memorial Sloan Kettering Cancer Center, New York, New York

EDMUND PRIBITKIN, MD
Professor and Academic Vice Chair, Department of Otolaryngology-Head and Neck Surgery, Jefferson University College of Medicine, Philadelphia, Pennsylvania

GREGORY RANDOLPH, MD, FACS, FACE
Division of Thyroid and Parathyroid Surgery, Department Otology and Laryngology, Massachusetts Eye and Ear Infirmary, Harvard Medical School; Division of Surgical Oncology, Massachusetts General Hospital, Boston, Massachusetts

DAVID W. SCHOPPY, MD, PhD
Division of Head and Neck Surgery, Department of Otolaryngology, Stanford University School of Medicine, Stanford, California

ASHOK R. SHAHA, MD
Head and Neck Service, Department of Surgery, Memorial Sloan Kettering Cancer Center, New York, New York

CHARALAMBOS SOLOMIDES, MD
Associate Professor, Director of Cytopathology; Department of Pathology, Jefferson University Hospital, Philadelphia, Pennsylvania

BRENDAN C. STACK Jr, MD, FACS, FACE
Professor and Chair, Department of Otolaryngology-Head and Neck Surgery, University of Arkansas for Medical Sciences, Little Rock, Arkansas

DAVID L. STEWARD, MD
Professor, Department of Otolaryngology–Head and Neck Surgery; Division of Endocrinology, Department of Medicine, University of Cincinnati College of Medicine, Cincinnati, Ohio

DAVID J. TERRIS, MD, FACS
Porubsky Professor and Chairman, Department of Otolaryngology, Georgia Regents University, Augusta, Georgia

GABRIEL J. TSAO, MD
Department of Otolaryngology–Head and Neck Surgery, University of California, San Francisco, San Francisco, California

RALPH P. TUFANO, MD, MBA, FACS
Charles W. Cummings MD Professor; Director, Division of Head and Neck Endocrine Surgery, Department of Otolaryngology-Head and Neck Surgery, Johns Hopkins Outpatient Center, The Johns Hopkins University School of Medicine, Baltimore, Maryland

MADALINA TULUC, MD
Assistant Professor, Department of Pathology, Jefferson University Hospital, Philadelphia, Pennsylvania

LINWAH YIP, MD
Assistant Professor of Endocrine Surgery and Surgical Oncology, Department of Surgery, University of Pittsburgh, Pittsburgh, Pennsylvania

Contents

nonpalpable lesions. This article discusses the indications, variations, and technical details of ultrasound-guided FNA.

Surgical Diagnosis: Frozen Section and the Extent of Surgery 519

Iain J. Nixon, Ashok R. Shaha, and Snehal G. Patel

This article outlines features of the biology of well differentiated thyroid cancer, and how these impact on systems of risk prediction. It covers salient points that the surgeon should consider from the clinical history and examination in the office, and outlines the procedures available for surgical management of thyroid cancer. The article then examines the choices that face thyroid surgeons both in relation to planning primary thyroid surgery and the approach to regional lymphadenectomy. In addition, key findings in the operating room are discussed in relation to their impact on decision making. Long-term outcomes are presented for patients following surgery.

Contemporary Surgical Techniques 529

William S. Duke, Katrina Chaung, and David J. Terris

Recent technologic advances have engendered alternative and innovative approaches to thyroid surgery aimed at reducing cosmetic sequelae. Minimally invasive techniques via small anterior cervical incisions hidden in natural skin creases and remote access approaches that eliminate anterior neck incisions entirely have emerged as viable options for patients who regard cosmesis as a priority. The safe application of these techniques to both benign and malignant thyroid disease has been evaluated.

Management of the Neck in Thyroid Cancer 545

David W. Schoppy and F. Christopher Holsinger

The management of regional lymph nodes in thyroid carcinoma is guided by preoperative evaluation, histologic subtype, and often a consideration of data for potential benefit and morbidity of a neck dissection. The goal of lymphadenectomy is complete surgical resection of grossly evident metastatic disease and the removal of regional lymph node groups at highest risk for microscopic disease. Surgery should achieve disease eradication but preserve voice, airway, swallowing, and parathyroid function. This article discusses recommendations for addressing cervical lymph nodes in thyroid carcinoma, discusses current literature regarding the common histologic subtype (papillary carcinoma), and details our operative approach.

Clinical Application of Molecular Testing of Fine-needle Aspiration Specimens in Thyroid Nodules 557

Linwah Yip and Robert L. Ferris

Thyroid cancer is the most common endocrine malignancy, and its incidence is increasing. Thyroid cancer is typically diagnosed during the evaluation of thyroid nodules. Although most thyroid nodules are benign, the challenge is to accurately and effectively identify malignant nodules. Understanding of genetic pathways involved in thyroid carcinogenesis has improved, and molecular testing techniques have become widespread

OTOLARYNGOLOGIC CLINICS OF NORTH AMERICA

FORTHCOMING ISSUES

October 2014
Common ENT Disorders in Children
Charles Bower and Gresham T. Richter, *Editors*

December 2014
Ear Implants
Colin L.W. Driscoll and Brian A. Neff, *Editors*

February 2015
Pediatric Head and Neck Masses
John P. Maddalozzo and Jeffrey Rastatter, *Editors*

RECENT ISSUES

June 2014
Robotic Surgery in Otolaryngology
Neil D. Gross and F. Chris Holsinger, *Editors*

April 2014
Headache in Otolaryngology: Rhinogenic and Beyond
Howard Levine and Michael Setzen, *Editors*

February 2014
Asthma: Screening, Diagnosis, and Management
Karen H. Calhoun, *Editor*

RELATED INTEREST

Surgical Pathology Clinics, Volume 7, Issue 4, December 2014
Endocrine Pathology
Peter Sadow, *Editor*

Correction

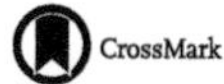

The name of author Fliippo Montevecchi MD was misspelled in the article "Transoral Robotic Sleep Surgery: The Obstructive Sleep Apnea-Hypopnea Syndrome," in the April 2014 issue of Otolaryngologic Clinics, "Robotic Surgery of the Head and Neck," edited by Neil Gross MD and Christopher Holsinger MD. The article is authored by Crawford JA; Montevecchi F; Vicini C; Magnuson JS.

Otolaryngol Clin N Am 47 (2014) xiii
http://dx.doi.org/10.1016/j.otc.2014.06.013
0030-6665/14/$ – see front matter

Preface

Thyroid Cancer: Current Diagnosis, Management, and Prognostication

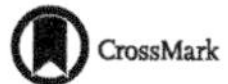

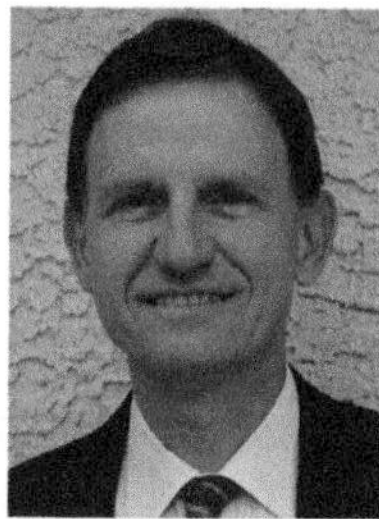

Robert L. Witt, MD, FACS
Editor

Winds of change are underway in the diagnosis, management, and prognostication of thyroid nodules. This issue of *Otolaryngologic Clinics of North America* is dedicated to the firmament of clinical evaluation and classic surgical approach to the thyroid nodule with a focus on the rapid evolution within the field.

A historic diagnostic leap was ushered in decades ago with fine-needle aspiration cytology (FNAC) for the palpable thyroid nodule. Benign FNAC eliminated the need for diagnostic thyroid surgery in many instances. FNAC less commonly makes a diagnosis of thyroid cancer. Indeterminate FNAC is an active area of surgical intervention, although only a relatively small percentage of the large number of diagnostic thyroid procedures have yielded a final diagnosis of cancer.

The next diagnostic leap has been the use of thyroid ultrasound that has led to refinement in characterizing suspicious features of many thyroid nodules and identification of impalpable thyroid nodules. Subsequent popularization of ultrasound-guided FNAC has led to the diagnosis of smaller and smaller thyroid nodules with cancer and accounts in large part to the swift rise in the reported incidence of thyroid cancer in North America and elsewhere.

One ongoing diagnostic challenge is the unfortunate circumstance of completion thyroidectomy in cases of indeterminate FNAC and frozen-section analysis that is proven to be cancer on final pathology several days after diagnostic thyroid lobectomy. A second more common challenge remains the high rate of diagnostic thyroid surgery for indeterminate nodules that is ultimately proved benign and in retrospect was unnecessary surgery for the patient. Fine-needle aspiration (FNA) with molecular alteration testing has high diagnostic specificity and positive predictive value. It holds considerable promise in reducing the need for completion thyroidectomy. FNA with

Otolaryngol Clin N Am 47 (2014) xv–xvi
http://dx.doi.org/10.1016/j.otc.2014.06.001

gene expression testing has high diagnostic sensitivity and negative predictive value. It portends to reduce the number of unnecessary diagnostic thyroid surgeries.

Fundamental to thyroid surgical management is an intimate understanding of thyroid, parathyroid, and neck anatomy, including neural and vascular structures. Technical innovations prompt us to compare time-honored classic open approaches with video-assisted, endoscopic, and robotic approaches. Extent of thyroid and neck surgery has long had forceful, sometimes opposing opinions. Molecular alteration testing will add fuel to the debate initially, but portends to lead to a personalized targeted surgical approach in the not too distant future.

Prognostication for survival and recurrence in patients with thyroid cancer has relied on a number of risk-stratification schemes. Molecular alteration testing is on the horizon to enhance prognostication for the individual patient.

Few fields in medicine rival the dynamism of modern thyroid diagnosis, management, and prognostication.

Robert L. Witt, MD, FACS
Head and Neck Multidisciplinary Clinic
Helen F. Graham Cancer Center
Christiana Care
4745 Ogletown-Stanton Road
MAP #1, Suite 112
Newark, DE 19713, USA

E-mail address:
RobertLWitt@gmail.com

Evidence-Based Evaluation of the Thyroid Nodule

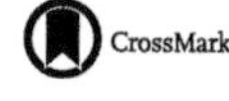

Louise Davies, MD, MS[a,b,c,*], Gregory Randolph, MD[d,e]

KEYWORDS

• Thyroid • Thyroid nodule • Thyroid cancer • Evaluation • Thyroid neoplasm risk

KEY POINTS

- Thyroid nodules are extraordinarily common; by age 90, virtually everyone has nodules.
- Ultrasound is the most valuable imaging study for making decisions about which nodules to biopsy.
- Nodules that are greater than 2 cm in size, that are entirely solid in composition, and that have microcalcifications are most likely to harbor a cancer.
- Molecular markers can help predict the presence of malignancy in cytologically indeterminate nodules, but markers do not accurately predict aggressiveness of cancers.
- Small papillary thyroid cancers can be safely observed in selected patients; discussions with patients should incorporate this option.

THE THYROID NODULE—SCOPE OF THE PROBLEM

Thyroid nodules are extraordinarily common. A key challenge for clinicians is to decide which ones require evaluation and intervention. Half of people age 50 or over with clinically normal thyroid glands and thyroid function have thyroid nodules, and by age 90, virtually everyone has nodules.[1] Thyroid cancer is commonly found at autopsy in

---

Authorship: Conception and design, acquisition of data, analysis, drafting of article (L. Davies); conception and design, critical revision of article (G. Randolph).
Disclaimers: The views expressed do not necessarily represent the views of the Department of Veterans Affairs, or the United States Government.
Sources of Support: The Department of Veterans Affairs.
Conflicts of Interest: No financial conflict of interest to declare.
[a] Department of Veterans Affairs Medical Center, VA Outcomes Group, 111B, 215 North Main Street, White River Junction, VT 05009, USA; [b] Section of Otolaryngology, Geisel School of Medicine at Dartmouth, Rope Ferry Road, Hanover, NH 03755, USA; [c] The Dartmouth Institute for Health Policy and Clinical Practice, 35 Centerra Parkway, Lebanon, NH 03766, USA; [d] Division of Thyroid and Parathyroid Surgery, Department Otology and Laryngology, Massachusetts Eye and Ear Infirmary, Harvard Medical School, 243 Charles Street, Boston, MA 02114, USA; [e] Division of Surgical Oncology, Massachusetts General Hospital, 55 Fuit Street, Boston, MA 02114, USA
* Corresponding author. VA Outcomes Group, 111B, 215 North Main Street, White River Junction, VT 05009.
E-mail address: louise.davies@va.gov

http://dx.doi.org/10.1016/j.otc.2014.04.008
0030-6665/14/$ – see front matter Published by Elsevier Inc.

individuals who have died of other causes, never having been detected in that patient's life. Estimates of cancer prevalence at autopsy are quite variable and depend largely on the method used to detect the cancers and geographic location, but range from a low of about 4% to a high of 36%.[1–5] Thus, thyroid cancers can be clinically insignificant for many patients. The workup and treatment can potentially expose the patient to the risks of treatment without the likelihood of any benefit. This challenging aspect of thyroid nodules has been recognized for some time, but the problem has been compounded in recent years by advances in and proliferation of imaging technology.

Advanced radiologic imaging rates (computed tomography [CT], magnetic resonance imaging [MRI], nuclear medicine, and ultrasound) have increased 3-fold since 1996.[6] These scans commonly reveal small, nonpalpable thyroid nodules, which in the past would never have been identified because they were too small to detect by palpation, and too small to cause symptoms to the patient. Because so many of these incidental thyroid findings are now being uncovered, a dramatic increase in the observed incidence of small thyroid cancers is being experienced.[7,8]

The increase in thyroid cancer incidence caused by this phenomenon is a problem for several reasons. First, patients are exposed to harm from what is ultimately unnecessary treatment. Second, these incidental findings unnecessarily create "patients with cancer" with all the attendant anxiety, surveillance needs, and financial ramifications.[9] Last, these patients affect the validity of studies designed to understand and mitigate the risks of death or recurrence from thyroid cancer by serving to falsely improve the results of clinical trials. With this in mind, the chief challenge to clinicians today is deciding which nodules require workup, and how aggressively to treat them. What follows is a review of the current evidence related to the approach to the patient with a nodule.

PATIENT PRESENTATION

When a patient comes to the office with a thyroid nodule, the mechanism of detection is of paramount importance and will determine what next steps should be taken (**Fig. 1**). A patient who presents with symptoms of tracheal or esophageal compression should raise concern for a malignancy, although large goiter and Hashimoto thyroiditis can also cause these types of symptoms. The clinician should inquire regarding symptoms related to change in ease of breathing, swallowing, and speech quality. In contrast, a mass that was first noticed by the patient but that is not otherwise causing symptoms will have a much broader differential diagnosis (**Table 1**). Although a rapid increase in size can signal malignancy, it can also signal hemorrhage into a benign neoplasm.

Today, many thyroid nodules come to attention through radiologic imaging studies. The nodules are subclinical—not causing any symptoms for the patient and generally not apparent on the physical examination. There are 2 main pathways of such radiologic detection—the first is through incidental detection on radiologic imaging studies done for other reasons, such as chest CT (obtained for cough, for example), neck MRI (performed after motor vehicle accident/suspected whiplash injury, for example), or carotid ultrasound. The second pathway is detection through a "diagnostic cascade" of nontargeted and sometimes inappropriate initial testing—for example, when a thyroid ultrasound is inappropriately ordered as part of a more general workup for weight gain, fatigue, or hair loss—and a thyroid nodule is found but is unrelated to the patient's presenting symptoms.[8] There are emerging data suggesting that traditional thyroid cancer risk factors, such as age, may be different for subclinical nodules that turn out to be papillary thyroid cancer on evaluation than for clinically apparent cancers, so obtaining a complete history is of even greater importance than in the past.[10]

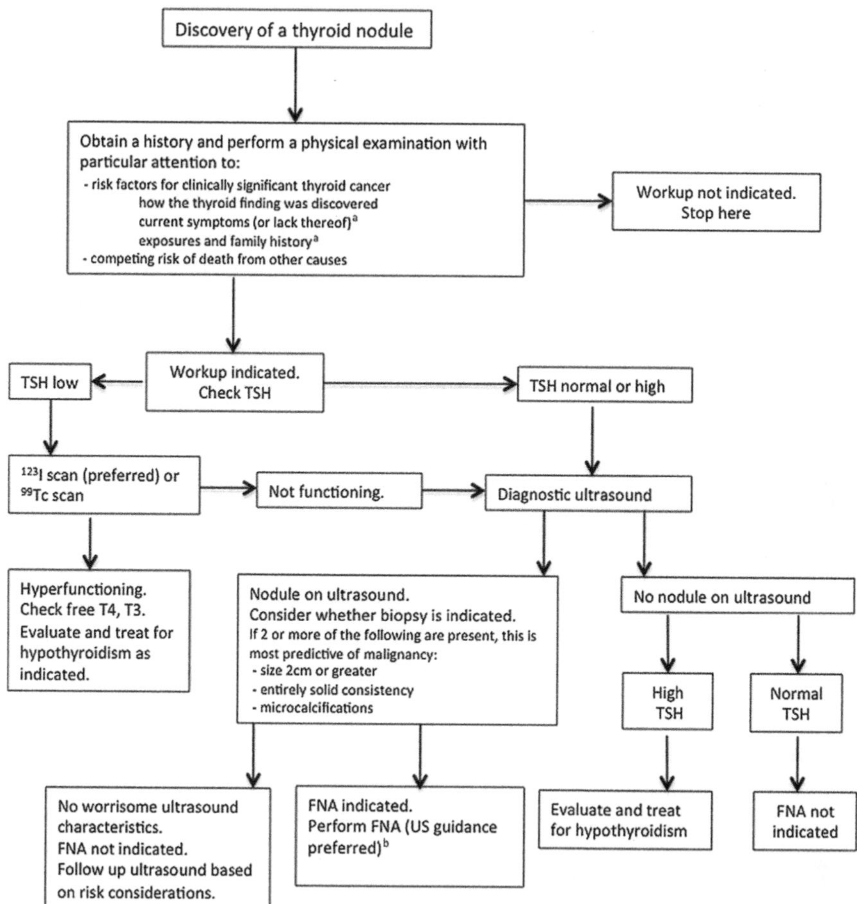

Fig. 1. Thyroid nodule evaluation algorithm based on current best available evidence. [a] See **Box 1, Table 2** for risk assessment details. [b] See **Table 3** for interpretation and recommendations for action based on FNA results. US, ultrasound.

On physical examination, a mass that is hard and fixed may indicate malignancy, but a mass may also be hard in patients with Hashimoto thyroiditis. The presence of palpable adenopathy should raise suspicions of malignancy. Lymph nodes may be biopsied if radiographically indeterminate as part of the initial workup.

Table 1
Differential diagnosis of the thyroid nodule

Benign	Malignant
Multinodular goiter	Papillary carcinoma (88%)
Hashimoto thyroidtis	Follicular carcinoma (9%)
Simple or hemorrhagic cyst	Hurthle cell (oxyphilic) type
Follicular adenoma	Medullary carcinoma (<2%)
Subacute thyroiditis	Anaplastic (<2%)
	Primary thyroid lymphoma (rare)
	Metastases from breast, renal cell, others (rare)

ASSESSMENT OF RISK FACTORS

Traditional risk factors for thyroid cancer in a thyroid nodule include age, gender, history of radiation exposure, family history of thyroid cancer, and cancer syndromes. Data refining the significance of these risks continue to evolve (**Box 1**).[11]

Age

It is often stated that the risk of finding cancer in a nodule is greater among patients who are less than age 30 or greater than age 60.[12] However, in one commonly quoted study, patients were only included if they were operated on, which limits its generalizability to the broader population of all people undergoing thyroid nodule evaluation. Furthermore, to be operated on, patients had to have both a cold nodule on scintigraphy and also a suspicious needle biopsy. Thus, the data from this study are not useful for predicting cancer risk in a patient who presents to a clinician without having had any workup performed.

Box 1
Risk factors for malignancy in a thyroid nodule

Risk factors

- Symptoms
  - Persistent hoarseness, dysphagia, or dysphonia
  - Lump is growing
- History
  - Radiation exposure before age 20:
    - Therapeutic irradiation
    - Advanced medical imaging (eg, CT scan/PET scan)
  - Family history
    - Multiple endocrine neoplasia type 2a and 2b
    - Medullary thyroid cancer
    - Nonmedullary thyroid cancer
    - Familial syndromes
      - Gardner syndrome (familial adenomatous polyposis)
      - Cowden syndrome (a PTEN hamartoma syndrome)
      - Pendred syndrome
      - Werner syndrome
      - Carney complex
- Physical findings
  - Male gender
  - Firm or hard consistency of the mass/nodule
  - Adenopathy of neck
  - Fixed to surrounding structures (rare)
  - Obvious voice, respiratory abnormality
  - Visible vocal cord abnormality

It may be more useful to consider age as a risk factor for *death* due to thyroid cancer. Understanding the risk of death allows one to decide about the utility of workup of a small nodule, because it allows assessment of the competing risks of death for a particular patient. Using this as a guide,[13] the prognosis of someone diagnosed with follicular cancer is worse if they are age 60 or over, and for medullary cancer, prognosis also begins to decrease precipitously at age 60. Age is not a strong determinant of prognosis for papillary cancer. Anaplastic histology has a very poor prognosis generally, but is much worse among people diagnosed at age 40 or over.

Gender

The risk of thyroid cancer has historically been stated to be higher in men than in women presenting with a thyroid nodule. Indeed, autopsy rates of subclinical thyroid cancer are slightly higher in men than in women.[1,3,5,14–16] However, the detected incidence of thyroid cancer is 3 times higher in women than in men.[17] This incidence is likely, in part, because men access health care less frequently than women in general, giving them fewer opportunities for a nodule to be discovered incidentally through physical examination.[18] In addition, male necks can be harder to examine than women's necks, so nodules are likely to be found when they are larger or more noticeable. Last, women at almost every age have slightly more nodules than men,[1] making them more likely to undergo workup than men. Thus, for a given individual presenting with a clinically apparent thyroid nodule, the likelihood of finding a cancer in the nodule is greater in a man than a woman.

Radiation Exposure

Data from long-term follow-up studies of Hiroshima and Nagasaki nuclear bomb survivors in Japan have recently been published. These studies show that the increased risk of thyroid cancer after a single large radiation exposure persists for at least 50 years. People exposed to 1 Gy or more from the bombings who were under the age of 20 have a 29% greater risk of developing thyroid cancer than for people of the same age who were not exposed.[19] The younger people were at the time of exposure, the greater the risk of developing a thyroid cancer; however, individuals who were older than age 20 at the time of the bombings have not demonstrated an elevated risk of thyroid cancer. The risk of thyroid cancer from lower radiation doses received over a long period of time (eg, from medical imaging) cannot be directly inferred from these data, because the mechanism of action is different. However, rates are expected to be lower than that described above.

In a recent cohort study of Australian children ages 0 to 19 followed for a mean of 9.5 years after one CT scan (~4.5-mSv radiation), there was a 24% increased risk of solid, leukemic, and lymphoid cancer in exposed children compared with children not so exposed. Subsequent CT scans incrementally increased the risk further, and the risk was greater for people exposed at younger ages, similar to the Japanese Hiroshima and Nagasaki data on one-time large exposures from the bombings.[20] A complete history should thus include a query about exposure to advanced medical imaging—such as CT or positron emission tomography (PET) scans—during childhood and adolescence.

Family History and Cancer Syndromes

Family history has long been recognized to be a risk factor for medullary thyroid cancer. It is also now increasingly recognized to be a risk for the other thyroid cancer histologies. Two recent studies, one from the United States and the other from northern

Europe, suggest about a 3-fold increased risk of developing nonmedullary thyroid cancer if a first-degree relative has had the diagnosis.[21,22]

Several familial and syndromic cancer disorders are associated with increased thyroid cancer risk. Persons with familial adenomatous polyposis (Gardner syndrome) are reported to have a 1% to 2% lifetime risk of developing thyroid cancer, with a mean age at diagnosis of 28 years.[23] This risk is just slightly greater than the current 1.1% lifetime risk of developing thyroid cancer in the in the United States.[24] More serious is Cowden syndrome, one of the phosphatase and tensin homologue (PTEN) hamartoma tumor syndromes, which confers increased risk of breast and thyroid cancers. The risk of thyroid cancer in patients with this syndrome is increased 38% compared with people without the syndrome.[25] In multiple endocrine neoplasia syndrome, types 2a and 2b are associated with medullary thyroid cancer.[26] Patients with Pendred syndrome (deafness, goiter, and iodine organification abnormalities), Werner syndrome (premature aging and abnormal growth), Carney complex (myxomas of heart and skin, lentigines of skin, and endocrine overactivity), isolated hyperparathyroidism or pheochromocytoma, marfanoid habitus, and mucosa neuromas are also potentially at increased risk of thyroid cancer.[27]

WORKUP OF THE THYROID NODULE

TSH and Other Laboratory Tests

After obtaining a history and physical examination, a decision will be made about whether to further pursue workup. The first step, if that workup is to be undertaken, is to obtain a result of thyroid stimulating hormone (TSH).[28,29] In a UK study, the rate of hyperthyroidism (15%) and hypothyroidism (2.3%) was higher in people undergoing nodule workup than the general population, so TSH assessment will allow identification of people with thyroid dysfunction requiring treatment regardless of the rest of the workup. In this same study, if the TSH was greater than 5.5, the odds of finding a thyroid malignancy on needle biopsy were 11 times greater than if the TSH was in the normal range.[30] A low TSH result should be followed by thyroid scintigraphy for workup. A normal TSH should be followed by needle biopsy if appropriate, and a high TSH should get a workup for hypothyroidism in addition to needle biopsy when indicated.

Obtaining a calcitonin level is not recommended in the United States for several reasons, although there is not uniformity in US guidelines.[28,31] Three major reasons given to omit calcitonin assessment are as follows:

1. There is a high false positive rate (59% or more) in some studies.[32]
2. Pentagastrin is not available in the United States for further stratifying cancer risk if a high basal calcitonin result is found.
3. The serum calcitonin cutoff levels for sporadic medullary thyroid cancer have not been agreed on.[33]

Measurement of serum antithyroid peroxidase antibodies is not necessary in the routine workup of a thyroid nodule. Although it may help define the patients with autoimmune thyroiditis, it does not necessarily obviate fine-needle aspiration (FNA) if a discrete nodule is present. Serum thyroglobulin measurements are also unnecessary. These levels can be elevated in both benign and malignant disease and vary by gender and age.

Scintigraphy

Scintigraphy has been largely replaced by ultrasound, but still has at least 2 roles: identifying hyperfunctioning nodules when a low TSH is found on initial testing, and to a limited extent, determining which nodule to sample in patients with multiple nodules. The latter indication has now been largely replaced by ultrasound assessment.

Scintigraphy can be performed using ^{123}I or technetium-99m pertechnetate. However, radioiodine is preferred, because about 5% of thyroid cancers will be missed by pertechentate in people with normal TSH.[34] Nonfunctioning ("cold," uptake less than surrounding tissues) nodules may warrant needle biopsy, depending on size and ultrasound characteristics. Autonomous nodules ("hot," uptake more than surrounding tissues) do not require needle biopsy, as they rarely harbor cancer.[35] If the nodule is functioning but not making enough thyroid hormone to suppress TSH, it may appear indeterminate on scintigraphy.

Indeterminate nodules may occur for the reason outlined above, but can also occur because, as a 2-dimensional image, abnormal tissue may have normal tissue superimposed on it. This abnormal tissue with superimposed normal tissue may be particularly true when nodules are less than 2 cm in size.[35] For the purpose of biopsy decisions, indeterminate nodules should be treated as though they are nonfunctioning.

Ultrasound

Thyroid ultrasound is the first choice of imaging studies for thyroid gland evaluation. Nodule size, detailed characteristics, anatomic location, and condition of nearby structures are all clearly delineated. Ultrasound has been shown to be more accurate than physical examination in detecting nodules.[36]

Ultrasound qualities of a nodule in isolation are not diagnostic of a malignancy, but they do indicate which nodules are more likely to harbor malignancy, and so can inform decision-making about nodule selection for biopsy.

Several ultrasound findings have been found to be associated with malignancy among patients brought to surgery after biopsy (**Table 2**). However, in a recent well-done case control study,[37] only 3 of the commonly cited characteristics were found to be the most useful:

1. Microcalcifications
2. Size greater than 2 cm
3. Nodules that are entirely solid composition

If 2 of these 3 characteristics were used as criteria for biopsy, then the positive likelihood ratio for finding a cancer was 7.1, and only 16 biopsies needed to be done for every cancer identified. This approach reduces unnecessary biopsies by 90%, while maintaining a low risk of cancer (5 per 1000 patients for whom biopsy is deferred). Interestingly, these findings are strikingly similar to an article published in 1974,

Table 2
Ultrasound characteristics of thyroid nodules and their associations with benign or malignant diagnosis

Benign	Malignant
Hyperechoic	Size 2 cm or greater
Peripheral vascularity	Entirely solid
Spongiform appearance	Microcalcifications
Comet tail shadowing	Hypoechoic
Purely cystic	Central vascularity
	Irregular margins
	Incomplete halo
	Nodule taller than wide

when there was less sophisticated technology available for nodule evaluation.[38] In that article, the following similar triad of findings were recommended as criteria for action:

1. Size greater than 2 to 2.5 cm
2. Solid nodule consistency by palpation
3. Evidence of microcalcification on plain radiograph

At that time, the detected incidence rates of thyroid cancer were much lower, but the mortality was the same as it is today, suggesting that the approach recommended in this most recent study would likely be sound and would not lead to in an increased risk of missing clinically important cancers.

Both the American Association of Clinical Endocrinologists (AACE) and the American Thyroid Association (ATA) guidelines suggest nodules as small as 5 mm might be biopsied and should be followed based on risk factors alone. However, using size alone as criteria is more likely to result in the detection of clinically unimportant cancers. Thus, for small nodules, the authors support a more measured approach that incorporates ultrasound characteristics into the decision-making process.

Large nodules also merit discussion. Some nodules are so large it has been asserted that they should be surgically removed without taking the extra step of biopsy. In an article published in 2007, among patients brought to surgery who had been diagnosed with nodules greater than 4 cm, needle biopsy results were frequently false negative. For this reason, they suggested that size alone might be used as criteria for surgical intervention in large nodules.[39] The authors think that because large nodules (~4 cm or greater) are less accurately assessed by FNA and because they often eventually affect speech and swallow function due to size, surgical intervention should be considered.

Needle Biopsy

Needle biopsy of the thyroid gland as a tool to decrease unnecessary surgery was first reported in 1973.[40] Several studies, both historic and recent, have confirmed its utility and success in lowering rates of unnecessary surgery.[41–44] The terminology surrounding cytologic diagnosis was standardized in 2009 with the introduction of the Bethesda criteria,[45] modeled after criteria developed for interpretation of Pap smears of the cervix.

The accepted classifications and the standard nomenclature are nondiagnostic, benign, atypia of undetermined significance or follicular lesion of undetermined significance (FLUS), follicular neoplasm, suspicious for malignancy, or malignant. Although the criteria have been useful as a standardized nomenclature, they have not improved the interrater reliability problems in thyroid cytology, which represents a particularly difficult problem in the atypical cells of uncertain significance (AUS)/FLUS category.[46] In particular, rates of FLUS category usage have been shown to vary from 2.5% to 28.6% across individual pathologists (**Table 3**). Furthermore, because many studies estimating FNA reliability in diagnosing cancer leave out the middle categories of uncertainty when making their calculations about sensitivity, specificity, and positive and negative predictive value, published results may not indicate the results seen in daily practice at a given institution.[47,48] Thus, for best results, each clinician should learn the reading practices typical of their institution and then calculate their own institution-specific likelihood of finding cancer in each type of biopsy result.

In many cases, there will be more than one nodule discovered during the ultrasound of the thyroid gland. The risk of malignancy is no lower or higher whether there are multiple nodules or a single nodule,[49,50] so the ATA guidelines suggest biopsy of those nodules preferentially that have the most worrisome ultrasound characteristics. The

Table 3
Thyroid needle biopsy

Classification Category	Possible Action
Nondiagnostic or unsatisfactory	Repeat ultrasound-guided biopsy, unless purely cystic.
Benign	Follow clinically. Consider repeat ultrasound to assess for growth in 6–18 mo if clinically indicated.
Atypia of undetermined significance Or Follicular lesion of undetermined significance	Repeat the needle biopsy. If results the same: Consider molecular testing Or Proceed to surgery based on clinical or ultrasound features.
Follicular neoplasm Or Suspicious for follicular neoplasm	Thyroid lobectomy.
Suspicious for malignancy	Lobectomy or thyroidectomy.
Malignant	Near total or total thyroidectomy.

Data from Refs.[28,31,45]

ATA 2009 Guidelines also suggest that if there are multiple nodules and *none* have characteristics indicative of malignancy, it is reasonable to biopsy the largest one. However, this recommendation was acknowledged to be based on expert opinion level "C." The authors think biopsy of nodules without ultrasound characteristics consistent with malignancy will result in unnecessary biopsies, exposing patients to a risk of harm with no expectation of benefit.[37]

Molecular Markers

Needle biopsy results that are read as "benign" or "malignant" provide clear data on which to make clinical decisions. Unfortunately, up to nearly a third of needle biopsies will be returned as cytologically indeterminate. In that setting, molecular markers that predict malignancy or define a benign nodule may provide additional clues about the presence or absence of malignancy in the nodule and have application in surgical decision-making. The key markers associated with thyroid cancer in FLUS samples are BRAF, RAS, RET/PTC, and PAX8/PPARγ. In a 2011 study, the presence of these findings in an FLUS lesion conferred a risk of malignancy of 88%.[51] This topic is extensively reviewed in other articles in this issue.

Published studies of molecular testing vary in their estimates of malignancy risk, and this is likely at least partly because of the evolving nature of the methods used to identify the mutations. For example, it was recently shown that 3 commonly used methods to test for BRAF resulted in quite different sensitivities for the mutation, varying from 54% to 80%, with the "mutant enrichment with 3′-modified oligonucleotide sequencing" method having the best sensitivity.[52]

Although molecular markers can assist in choosing indeterminate lesions for surgical intervention, the value of the markers for prognostication of known papillary thyroid cancers is less clear. Specifically, several recent studies performed in different patient populations have not consistently found an association between the presence of BRAF V600e and the risk of recurrence, mortality, or papillary thyroid cancer aggressiveness.[53–55] Overall, tumor pathologic features continue to be most indicative of prognosis and therefore most clinically useful. Based on these data, molecular testing of needle biopsy specimens read as malignant will not add useful information to the therapeutic decision-making process.

CLOSING THOUGHTS ABOUT THYROID NODULE EVALUATION

Risk of Death for the Patient Found to Have a Thyroid Cancer

The point of evaluating a patient with a thyroid nodule is to determine whether a cancer is present. It is important to remember that, although everyone fears cancer, the outlook for patients diagnosed with papillary thyroid cancer, which is about 88% of thyroid cancers diagnosed in the United States, is excellent. The 20-year survival for papillary thyroid cancer of any size confined to the thyroid gland at the time of diagnosis is 99%.[56] For some patients, their competing risk of death from their other illnesses will be much greater, making workup of a thyroid nodule of lower utility to them. For those without competing illnesses, survival is so good that treatment decisions for small, incidentally detected papillary cancers should be made with consideration of the quality of life effects of each intervention chosen—including the decision to workup a small, incidentally detected thyroid nodule. Mortality in the United States due to thyroid cancer is low and has been stable for more than 30 years, despite recent trends in treatment toward increased aggressiveness, such as total thyroidectomy rather than lobectomy, and most recently the addition of prophylactic central neck dissection. At a rate of 0.5 per 100,000 people, the mortality due to thyroid cancer is about the same as it is for tuberculosis—that is, very rare.

Active Monitoring of Small Nodules

Not every thyroid nodule requires biopsy. For nodules falling outside the criteria for biopsy, it is reasonable to do follow-up ultrasound at intervals decided on in conjunction with the patient. Nodules can enlarge or become smaller over time, and there are good data to suggest that immediate action on thyroid cancer may not always be required, particularly when the nodules are small at the time of discovery.[56,57]

In recent years, selected small cancers have been observed rather than operated on immediately, and among those that grow or spread, surgical salvage has been successful,[57] which means that delaying treatment will not necessarily present a problem for patients. These facts should be part of the mental algorithm used when talking with patients about the decision to evaluate a thyroid nodule.

For the less common cancers, follicular, medullary, and anaplastic, the survival figures are different, and the prognosis is poorer. These cancers are dealt with in subsequent sections of this publication. Although the risks due to these cancers should also be part of the decision-making process in thyroid nodule evaluation, they are much less common; follicular cancers represent about 9% of all thyroid cancers, and anaplastic and medullary together account for 2%.[24]

Limitations of Existing Guidelines on Thyroid Nodule Management

Historic guidelines for thyroid nodule evaluation were designed for nodules found by palpation or because of symptoms experienced by the patient. Today, clinicians are increasingly faced with incidentally identified thyroid findings, but available guidelines do not yet explicitly address the emerging idea that incidentally identified nodules may be fundamentally different in their risk profile from those that are identified by a clinician or by patient symptoms.

Furthermore, although the ATA Guidelines for the management of thyroid nodules, published in 2009,[28] were based on an extensive reference search, the writers did not have available to them any studies that could strictly support an "A" recommendation rating for any of the nodule evaluation actions—the studies have not been done. Thus, all data available to make recommendations about thyroid nodule management are based on lower level data, indicating only an indirect effect on improving outcomes (grade B evidence) or lower.[58]

Although guidelines can help clinicians decide which tests to order, the decision of when to pursue workup will lie with the clinician and patient, who must make the decision together, understanding the risks and benefits of both pursuing and holding off on nodule evaluation. Summarized here is the current evidence regarding thyroid nodule and their management to aid joint decision-making about which nodules should be worked up and treated, which should be actively monitored, and which can be safely left without further intervention.

REFERENCES

1. Mortensen JD, Woolner LB, Bennett WA. Gross and microscopic findings in clinically normal thyroid glands. J Clin Endocrinol Metab 1955;15(10):1270–80.
2. Harach HR, Franssila KO. Occult papillary carcinoma of the thyroid appearing as lung metastasis. Arch Pathol Lab Med 1984;108(7):529–30.
3. Martinez-Tello FJ, Martinez-Cabruja R, Fernandez-Martin J, et al. Occult carcinoma of the thyroid. A systematic autopsy study from Spain of two series performed with two different methods. Cancer 1993;71(12):4022–9.
4. Tanriover O, Comunoglu N, Eren B, et al. Occult papillary thyroid carcinoma: prevalence at autopsy in Turkish people. Eur J Cancer Prev 2011;20(4):308–12.
5. Lang W, Borrusch H, Bauer L. Occult carcinomas of the thyroid. Evaluation of 1,020 sequential autopsies. Am J Clin Pathol 1988;90(1):72–6.
6. Smith-Bindman R, Miglioretti DL, Johnson E, et al. Use of diagnostic imaging studies and associated radiation exposure for patients enrolled in large integrated health care systems, 1996-2010. JAMA 2012;307(22):2400–9.
7. Davies L, Welch HG. Increasing incidence of thyroid cancer in the United States, 1973-2002. JAMA 2006;295(18):2164–7.
8. Davies L, Ouellette M, Hunter M, et al. The increasing incidence of small thyroid cancers: where are the cases coming from? Laryngoscope 2010;120(12):2446–51.
9. Ramsey S, Blough D, Kirchhoff A, et al. Washington State cancer patients found to be at greater risk for bankruptcy than people without a cancer diagnosis. Health Aff (Millwood) 2013;32(6):1143–52.
10. Ito Y, Miyauchi A, Kobayashi K, et al. Prognosis and growth activity depend on patient age in clinical and subclinical papillary thyroid carcinoma [review]. Endocr J 2014;61(3):205–13.
11. Alexander E. Evaluation and management of thyroid nodules. 2nd edition. Philadelphia: Elsevier Saunders; 2012.
12. Belfiore A, La Rosa GL, La Porta GA, et al. Cancer risk in patients with cold thyroid nodules: relevance of iodine intake, sex, age, and multinodularity. Am J Med 1992;93(4):363–9.
13. Gilliland FD, Hunt WC, Morris DM, et al. Prognostic factors for thyroid carcinoma. A population-based study of 15,698 cases from the Surveillance, Epidemiology and End Results (SEER) program 1973-1991. Cancer 1997;79(3):564–73.
14. Harach HR, Franssila KO, Wasenius VM. Occult papillary carcinoma of the thyroid. A "normal" finding in Finland. A systematic autopsy study. Cancer 1985;56(3):531–8.

15. Ottino A, Pianzola HM, Castelletto RH. Occult papillary thyroid carcinoma at autopsy in La Plata, Argentina. Cancer 1989;64(2):547–51.
16. Solares CA, Penalonzo MA, Xu M, et al. Occult papillary thyroid carcinoma in postmortem species: prevalence at autopsy. Am J Otol 2005;26(2):87–90.
17. Davies L, Welch HG. Current thyroid cancer trends in the United States. JAMA Otolaryngol Head Neck Surg 2014;140(4):317–22.
18. Verbrugge LM. Sex differentials in health. Public Health Rep 1982;97(5): 417–37.
19. Furukawa K, Preston D, Funamoto S, et al. Long-term trend of thyroid cancer risk among Japanese atomic-bomb survivors: 60 years after exposure. Int J Cancer 2013;132(5):1222–6.
20. Mathews JD, Forsythe AV, Brady Z, et al. Cancer risk in 680,000 people exposed to computed tomography scans in childhood or adolescence: data linkage study of 11 million Australians. BMJ 2013;346:f2360.
21. Oakley GM, Curtin K, Pimentel R, et al. Establishing a familial basis for papillary thyroid carcinoma using the utah population database. JAMA Otolaryngol Head Neck Surg 2013;139(11):1171–4.
22. Fallah M, Pukkala E, Tryggvadottir L, et al. Risk of thyroid cancer in first-degree relatives of patients with non-medullary thyroid cancer by histology type and age at diagnosis: a joint study from five Nordic countries. J Med Genet 2013; 50(6):373–82.
23. Septer S, Slowik V, Morgan R, et al. Thyroid cancer complicating familial adenomatous polyposis: mutation spectrum of at-risk individuals. Hered Cancer Clin Pract 2013;11(1):13.
24. Cancer Fast Stats National Cancer Institute. Available at: http://seer.cancer.gov/faststats/. Accessed November 24, 2013.
25. Bubien V, Bonnet F, Brouste V, et al. High cumulative risks of cancer in patients with PTEN hamartoma tumour syndrome. J Med Genet 2013;50(4):255–63.
26. Gertner ME, Kebebew E. Multiple endocrine neoplasia type 2. Curr Treat Options Oncol 2004;5(4):315–25.
27. Richards ML. Familial syndromes associated with thyroid cancer in the era of personalized medicine. Thyroid 2010;20(7):707–13.
28. Cooper DS, Doherty GM, Haugen BR, et al. Revised American Thyroid Association management guidelines for patients with thyroid nodules and differentiated thyroid cancer. Thyroid 2009;19(11):1167–214.
29. National Comprehensive Care Network Guidelines for Thyroid Cancer. 2013.
30. Boelaert K, Horacek J, Holder RL, et al. Serum thyrotropin concentration as a novel predictor of malignancy in thyroid nodules investigated by fine-needle aspiration. J Clin Endocrinol Metab 2006;91(11):4295–301.
31. Gharib H, Papini E, Paschke R, et al. American Association of Clinical Endocrinologists, Associazione Medici Endocrinologi, and European Thyroid Association Medical guidelines for clinical practice for the diagnosis and management of thyroid nodules: executive summary of recommendations. Endocr Pract 2010;16(3): 468–75.
32. Castro MR, Gharib H. Continuing controversies in the management of thyroid nodules. Ann Intern Med 2005;142(11):926–31.
33. Giovanella L, Imperiali M, Ferrari A, et al. Thyroid volume influences serum calcitonin levels in a thyroid-healthy population: results of a 3-assay, 519 subjects study. Clin Chem Lab Med 2012;50(5):895–900.
34. Reschini E, Ferrari C, Castellani M, et al. The trapping-only nodules of the thyroid gland: prevalence study. Thyroid 2006;16(8):757–62.

35. Nelson RL, Wahner HW, Gorman CA. Rectilinear thyroid scanning as a predictor of malignancy. Ann Intern Med 1978;88(1):41–4.
36. Ezzat S, Sarti DA, Cain DR, et al. Thyroid incidentalomas. Prevalence by palpation and ultrasonography. Arch Intern Med 1994;154(16):1838–40.
37. Smith-Bindman R, Lebda P, Feldstein VA, et al. Risk of thyroid cancer based on thyroid ultrasound imaging characteristics: results of a population-based study. J Intern Med 2013;173(19):1788–95.
38. Greenspan FS. Thyroid nodules and thyroid cancer. West J Med 1974;121(5): 359–65.
39. McCoy KL, Jabbour N, Ogilvie JB, et al. The incidence of cancer and rate of false-negative cytology in thyroid nodules greater than or equal to 4 cm in size. Surgery 2007;142(6):837–44 [discussion: 844.e1–3].
40. Crile G Jr, Hawk WA Jr. Aspiration biopsy of thyroid nodules. Surg Gynecol Obstet 1973;136(2):241–5.
41. Kolendorf K, Hansen JB, Engberg L, et al. Fine needle and open biopsy in thyroid disorders. Acta Chir Scand 1975;141(1):20–3.
42. Colacchio TA, LoGerfo P, Feind CR. Fine needle cytologic diagnosis of thyroid nodules. Review and report of 300 cases. Am J Surg 1980;140(4):568–71.
43. Hamberger B, Gharib H, Melton LJ 3rd, et al. Fine-needle aspiration biopsy of thyroid nodules. Impact on thyroid practice and cost of care. Am J Med 1982; 73(3):381–4.
44. Van den Bruel A, Francart J, Dubois C, et al. Regional variation in thyroid cancer incidence in Belgium is associated with variation in thyroid imaging and thyroid disease management. J Clin Endocrinol Metab 2013;98(10):4063–71.
45. Cibas ES, Ali SZ, NCI Thyroid FNA State of the Science Conference. The Bethesda system for reporting thyroid cytopathology. Am J Clin Pathol 2009; 132(5):658–65.
46. Layfield LJ, Morton MJ, Cramer HM, et al. Implications of the proposed thyroid fine-needle aspiration category of "follicular lesion of undetermined significance": a five-year multi-institutional analysis. Diagn Cytopathol 2009;37(10):710–4.
47. Wong LQ, Baloch ZW. Analysis of the Bethesda system for reporting thyroid cytopathology and similar precursor thyroid cytopathology reporting schemes. Adv Anat Pathol 2012;19(5):313–9.
48. Lewis CM, Chang KP, Pitman M, et al. Thyroid fine-needle aspiration biopsy: variability in reporting. Thyroid 2009;19(7):717–23.
49. Marqusee E, Benson CB, Frates MC, et al. Usefulness of ultrasonography in the management of nodular thyroid disease. Ann Intern Med 2000;133(9):696–700.
50. Deandrea M, Mormile A, Veglio M, et al. Fine-needle aspiration biopsy of the thyroid: comparison between thyroid palpation and ultrasonography. Endocr Pract 2002;8(4):282–6.
51. Nikiforov YE, Ohori NP, Hodak SP, et al. Impact of mutational testing on the diagnosis and management of patients with cytologically indeterminate thyroid nodules: a prospective analysis of 1056 FNA samples. J Clin Endocrinol Metab 2011;96(11):3390–7.
52. Lee ST, Kim SW, Ki CS, et al. Clinical implication of highly sensitive detection of the BRAF V600E mutation in fine-needle aspirations of thyroid nodules: a comparative analysis of three molecular assays in 4585 consecutive cases in a BRAF V600E mutation-prevalent area. J Clin Endocrinol Metab 2012;97(7):2299–306.
53. Xing M, Alzahrani AS, Carson KA, et al. Association between BRAF V600E mutation and mortality in patients with papillary thyroid cancer. JAMA 2013; 309(14):1493–501.

54. Ito Y, Yoshida H, Kihara M, et al. BRAF Mutation analysis in papillary thyroid carcinoma: is it useful for all patients? World J Surg 2014;38(3):679–87.
55. Gouveia C, Can NT, Bostrom A, et al. Lack of association of BRAF mutation with negative prognostic indicators in papillary thyroid carcinoma: the University of California, San Francisco, experience. JAMA Otolaryngol Head Neck Surg 2013;139(11):1164–70.
56. Davies L, Welch HG. Thyroid cancer survival in the United States: observational data from 1973 to 2005. Arch Otolaryngol Head Neck Surg 2010;136(5):440–4.
57. Ito Y, Miyauchi A, Kihara M, et al. Patient age is significantly related to the progression of papillary microcarcinoma of the thyroid under observation. Thyroid 2014;24(1):27–34.
58. Dietlein M, Verburg FA, Luster M, et al. One should not just read what one believes: the nearly irresolvable issue of producing truly objective, evidence-based guidelines for the management of differentiated thyroid cancer. Eur J Nucl Med Mol Imaging 2011;38(5):793–8.

Thyroid Cytology

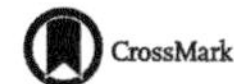

Madalina Tuluc, MD*, Charalambos Solomides, MD

KEYWORDS

• Cytopathology • Bethesda • Immunohistochemistry • Follicular • Atypia
• Carcinoma • Panels

KEY POINTS

- This article reviews the Bethesda System for Reporting Thyroid Cytology, with the diagnostic criteria for atypical and indeterminate categories reviewed.
- Having a unified way of reporting thyroid cytopathology is important for pathologists and clinicians alike.
- Although significant progress has been made in the discovery of new immunohistochemistry and molecular markers that indicate malignancy, no test can be used as stand-alone test in the diagnosis of thyroid malignancy.
- Various immunohistochemistry and molecular panels have entered the daily practice, either as a rule-in or as rule-out malignancy.
- These are commercially available panels with high positive or negative predictive value in detecting malignancy but more work is necessary.

INTRODUCTION

It is estimated that 4% to 7% of the adult population in the United States has a clinically palpable nodule, a number that increases significantly when imaging studies of the neck region performed for other indications are included. Combined incidence of clinically palpable and incidentally discovered nodules reaches 50% of the adult population of the United States.

In this context, over the past few decades, fine-needle aspiration (FNA) has developed as the most reliable and cost-effective method for the evaluation of a thyroid nodule, and it became the standard of care for the initial work-up of patients. Because of the extremely large number of benign thyroid nodules relative to malignant ones, FNA is used not only as a diagnostic test but also, in many cases, primarily as a screening test, which is used in conjunction with clinical findings and family history to guide patient management. FNA reduces unnecessary surgery for patients with benign nodules and triages patients with malignant nodules for surgical intervention.

Department of Pathology, Jefferson University Hospital, 132S 10th Street, Main Building, Philadelphia, PA 19107, USA
* Corresponding author.
E-mail address: madalina.tuluc@jefferson.edu

Otolaryngol Clin N Am 47 (2014) 475–489
http://dx.doi.org/10.1016/j.otc.2014.04.011
0030-6665/14/$ – see front matter

The goal of FNA is to provide pathologists with an adequate specimen that allows a meaningful interpretation. This implies a specimen with enough cellularity to yield a specific diagnosis and to minimize the number of false-negative results. Adequacy criteria are abundant in the literature; in the authors' practice, criteria suggested by the Bethesda System for Reporting Thyroid Cytology are used (ie, presence of at least 6 groups of well-preserved follicular cells with more than 10 cells per cluster). Generally, 2 to 3 passes with on-site adequacy evaluation by a cytopathologist are enough for an adequate specimen. Cellularity/adequacy is dependent not only on the technique of the aspirator but also on the inherent nature of the lesion (solid vs cystic).

In general, FNA results fall into 1 of 4 major diagnostic categories, with the relative frequency of diagnosis in parentheses: benign (70%), indeterminate or suspicious (10%–15%), malignant (5%), and nondiagnostic/unsatisfactory (10%–15%).[1]

It is critical that the cytopathology diagnosis is precise, unambiguous, and clinically helpful. In the past, terminology for thyroid FNA has varied significantly from one laboratory to another, creating confusion and preventing sharing of clinically meaningful data among multiple institutions.[2,3] To address the terminology and to establish strict diagnostic criteria for thyroid FNA samples, the Bethesda System for Reporting Thyroid Cytopathology established in 2008 offers a 6-category scheme, with the predicted probability of malignancy increasing from category II to VI: Bethesda I—nondiagnostic/unsatisfactory, Bethesda II—benign, Bethesda III—atypia of undetermined significance (AUS) or follicular lesion of undetermined significance (FLUS), Bethesda IV—follicular neoplasm or suspicious for follicular neoplasm (FN/SFN), Bethesda V—suspicious for malignancy (SFM), and Bethesda VI—malignant.

The indeterminate categories (Bethesda III to V) have an approximate cancer risk of 5% to 15%, 15% to 30%, and 60% to 75%, respectively.[2,4,5]

The goal of this article is to provide nonpathology clinicians with a summary of the most important concepts and categories of the Bethesda System for Reporting Thyroid Cytology and briefly describe the main cytologic criteria for the most common benign and malignant thyroid lesions.

NONDIAGNOSTIC SPECIMEN

The Bethesda I (nondiagnostic/unsatisfactory) category describes a specimen that fails to meet the adequacy criteria. The following scenarios describe nondiagnostic cases: fewer than 6 groups of well-preserved, well-stained follicular cells; poorly prepared, poorly stained, or obscured follicular cells (excessively bloody specimens); cyst fluid with or without histiocytes; and fewer than 6 groups of 10 follicular cells (**Fig. 1**).[4]

There are a few points that should be emphasized in this category. Adequacy criteria apply only to follicular cells and exclude macrophages or inflammatory cells. Therefore, in inflammatory conditions of the thyroid, such as lymphocytic thyroiditis, abscess, and granulomatous thyroiditis, follicular cells may be sparse and there is no minimum requirement for adequacy for follicular cells when inflammation predominates.

Cases of solid nodules with cytologic atypia—if the sample contains significant cytologic atypia—are never considered nondiagnostic. A comment describing scant cellularity is usually inserted in the report.

BENIGN THYROID LESIONS

The Bethesda II (benign) category includes benign follicular nodules and thyroiditis.

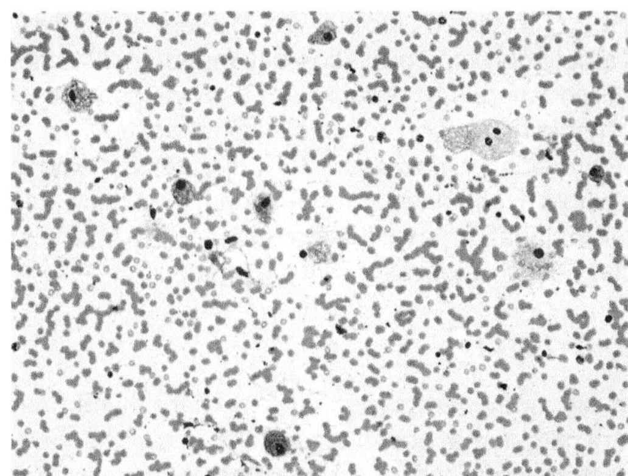

Fig. 1. Nondiagnostic specimen. Cyst fluid only. Few macrophages, rare inflammatory cells, and blood. There is no evidence of colloid or of follicular cells (Diff-Quik ×20).

Benign Follicular Nodule

Benign follicular nodule encompasses entities that are classified histologically as nodules in nodular goiter, hyperplastic (adenomatoid) nodule, colloid nodules, and nodules in Graves disease and is the most commonly encountered entity in Bethesda II category.[4,5] A specimen from a nodular goiter should have abundant colloid, follicular cells with small nuclei; smooth nuclear membrane; and fine even chromatin; forming monolayers; Hürthle cells; and macrophages (**Fig. 2**). The cellularity of such specimen can vary. Nodular goiters have usually moderate cellularity, but when they undergo cystic degeneration, the epithelial cellularity decreases and abundant macrophages are present. The hyperplastic (adenomatoid) nodule shares the same cytologic features with nodular goiter but the cellularity is much higher. Colloid nodule consists predominantly of colloid and, therefore, the FNA specimen is hypocellular with abundant colloid. An aspirate from a Graves disease nodule is hypercellular, with follicular cells showing colloid suds or fire flares (cytoplasmic vacuoles with colloid), Hürthle cell metaplasia, and scant colloid.

Thyroiditis

Lymphocytic thyroiditis, granulomatous thyroiditis, and acute thyroiditis are the other entities included in Bethesda II (benign) category. The cytologic features of

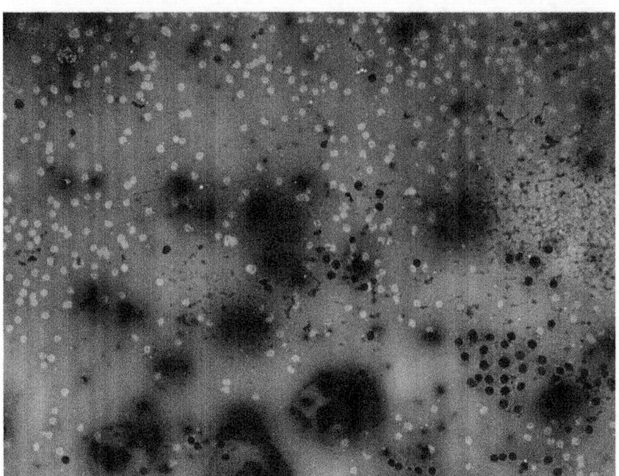

Fig. 2. Benign follicular nodule. Nodular goiter. Follicular cells in monolayers in the background of abundant colloid and few macrophages (Diff-Quik ×20).

lymphocytic (Hashimoto) thyroiditis include monolayers of Hürthle and follicular cells in a background of a polymorphic population of lymphocytes. Colloid should be scant (**Fig. 3**). The recommendation is to report such findings as "consistent with lymphocytic (Hashimoto) thyroiditis *in the proper clinical context*."[4] The cytologic features of granulomatous thyroiditis include scant follicular cells, mixed inflammatory cells, collections of epithelioid histiocytes (granulomas), multinucleated giant cells, and degenerated cellular material. An aspirate from an acute thyroiditis shows many neutrophils, few follicular cells, histiocytes, and bacteria.

MALIGNANT THYROID LESIONS

The Bethesda VI (malignant) category includes primary thyroid neoplasms (papillary carcinoma, medullary carcinoma, poorly differentiated carcinoma, and anaplastic carcinoma) as well as lymphoma and various metastatic tumors. In this category are included samples for which all criteria for malignancy are met and a diagnosis of malignancy can be established with certainty.

Papillary Carcinoma

The cytologic specimen from a papillary thyroid carcinoma (PTC) is usually hypercellular, with many follicular cells in monolayers and papillary formations. The nuclei are enlarged, oval-shaped, and pale with powdery chromatin, distinct nucleoli, nuclear grooves, and nuclear inclusions. There are also multinucleated giant cells and psammoma bodies. The amount of colloid is variable (**Figs. 4** and **5**). In addition to the classic PTC, there are several architectural and cytologic variants (follicular, macrofollicular, cystic, oncocytic, Warthin-like, tall cell, and columnar cell); all these variants have the essential nuclear features of PTC.[4–6]

Medullary Carcinoma

The cytologic features of medullary carcinoma include moderate to high cellularity, discohesive and loosely cohesive plasmacytoid or spindle cell, granular (salt-and-pepper) nuclear chromatin, and frayed cytoplasmic borders. Amyloid is usually present (**Figs. 6** and **7**). The neoplastic cells are positive for calcitonin and negative for thyroglobulin.[4,6]

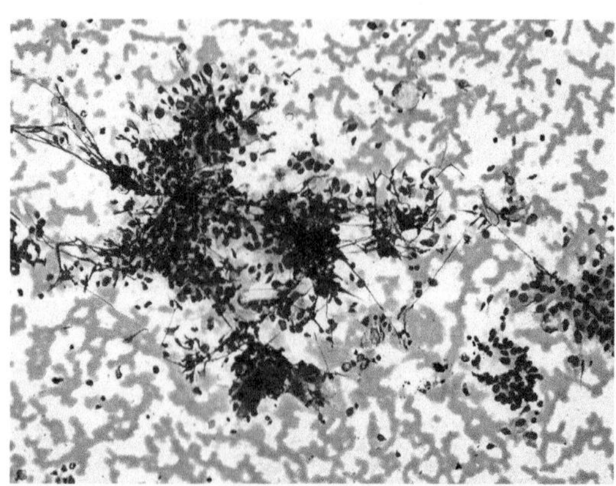

Fig. 3. Lymphocytic (Hashimoto) thyroiditis in the proper clinical context. Hürthle cell and follicular cells admixed with lymphocytes and lymphoid tangles (crushing lymphocyte artifact) (Diff-Quik ×20).

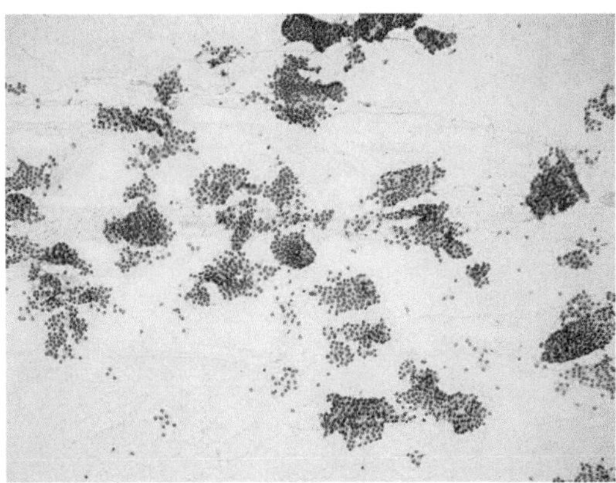

Fig. 4. PTC. Hypercellular specimen with monolayers and papillary formations of follicular cells (Papanicolau stain [PAP] ×10).

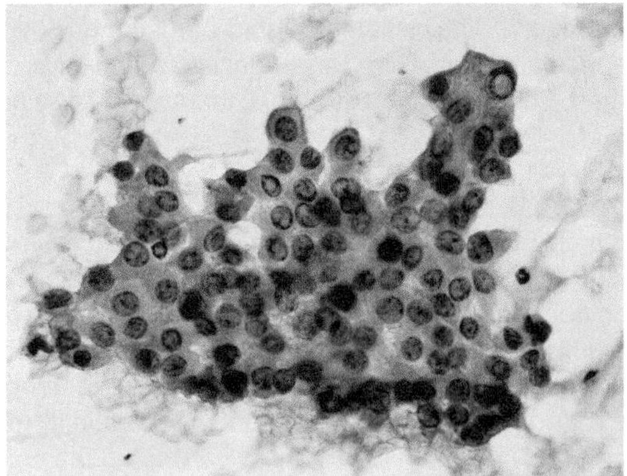

Fig. 5. PTC. Higher magnification showing nuclear enlagement, nuclear grooves, and nuclear inclusions (PAP ×60).

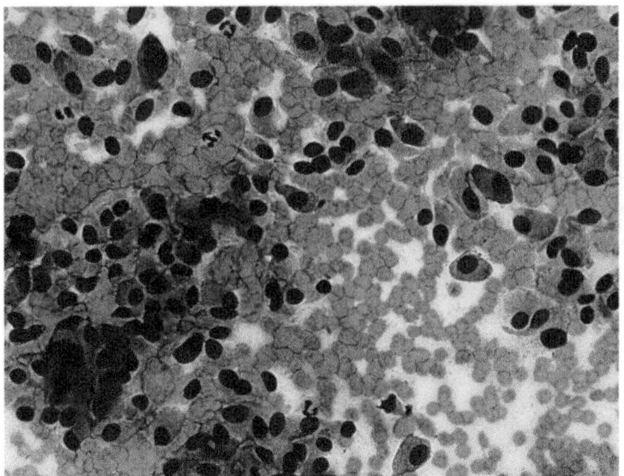

Fig. 6. Medullary carcinoma. Hypercellular specimen with plasmacytoid and spindle-shaped malignant cells (Diff-Quik ×40).

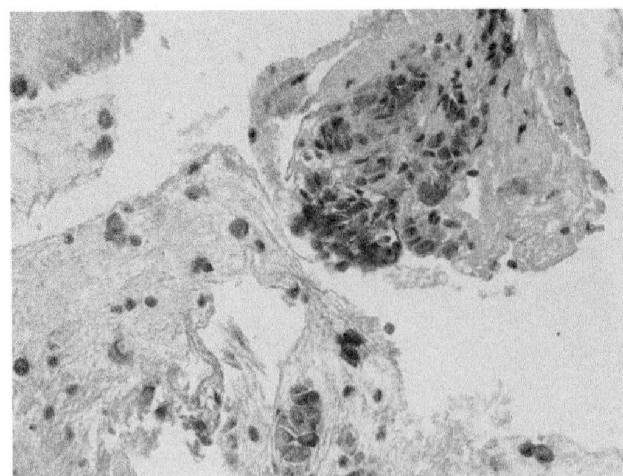

Fig. 7. Medullary carcinoma. Immunochistochemical stain for calcitonin; the malignant cells are positive (cell block ×20).

Poorly Differentiated Carcinoma

The specimen from a poorly differentiated thyroid carcinoma is hypercellular; has an insular, solid, or trabecular architecture; and consists of follicular cells with high nuclear/cytoplasmic ratio. There are nuclear atypia, increase mitotic activity, and necrosis (**Fig. 8**).[4,7]

Undifferentiated Anaplastic Carcinoma

The cytologic specimen from an anaplastic thyroid carcinoma is hypercellular and consists of malignant cells with enlarged, irregular, pleomorphic nuclei, in clusters and discohesive, including giant multinucleated and spindle-shaped tumor cells in a background of acute inflammation. Increased mitotic activity and necrosis are present. These tumor cells are negative for the usual thyroid markers, thyroglobulin and throid transcription factor 1, and they are positive for pancytokeratin (**Figs. 9** and **10**).[4,6]

Lymphoma

A majority of lymphomas involving the thyroid are secondary. Primary lymphomas are usually non-Hodgkin B-cell lymphomas (NHLs) and in approximately two-thirds of the

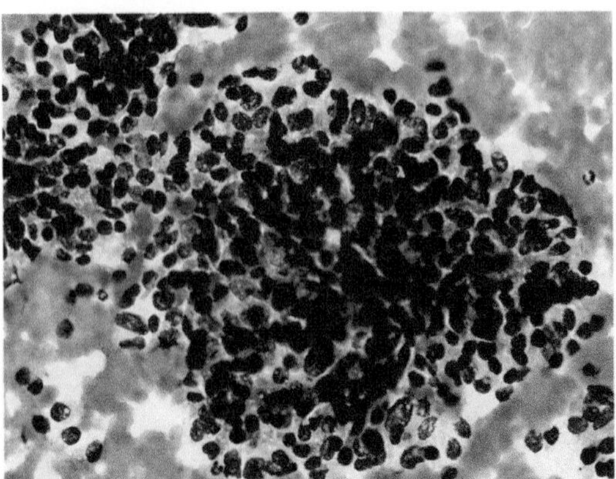

Fig. 8. Poorly differentiated thyroid carcinoma. Follicular cells with nuclear atypia in crowded insular arrangement (Diff-Quik ×40).

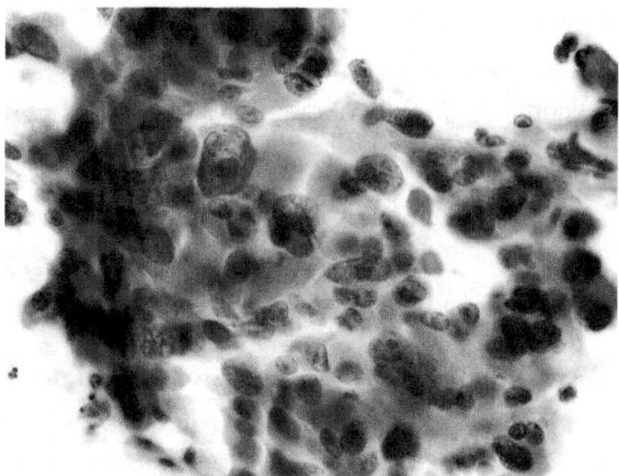

Fig. 9. Undifferentiated anaplastic thyroid carcinoma. Malignant cells with enlarged, irregular, pleomorphic nuclei, in clusters, including giant tumor cells (PAP ×40).

cases associated with Hashimoto thyroiditis.[4,8] Lymphomas represent approximately 5% of all thyroid neoplasms. The most common NHLs involving the thyroid are diffuse large B-cell lymphoma (DLBL) and extranodal marginal zone B-cell lymphoma. The aspirate from a lymphoma involving the thyroid is hypercellular and consists of either a monomorphic population of large atypical lymphoid cells (DLBL) or a mixture of small, intermediate, and large lymphoid cells that require immunophenotyping studies for diagnosis. It is strongly recommended that when the differential diagnosis at the time of the adequacy evaluation includes lymphoma, a separate sample from the FNA be sent to flow cytometry.

Metastatic Tumors to the Thyroid

Metastatic tumors to the thyroid are uncommon but do exist. The most common tumors metastasize to the thyroid are from lung, breast, skin (melanoma), colon, and kidney.[4,9] Direct extension from tumors from pharynx, larynx, esophagus, nearby lymph nodes, and the mediastinum also exist. The challenge to cytopathologists is to be able to recognize these tumors in a thyroid FNA specimen.

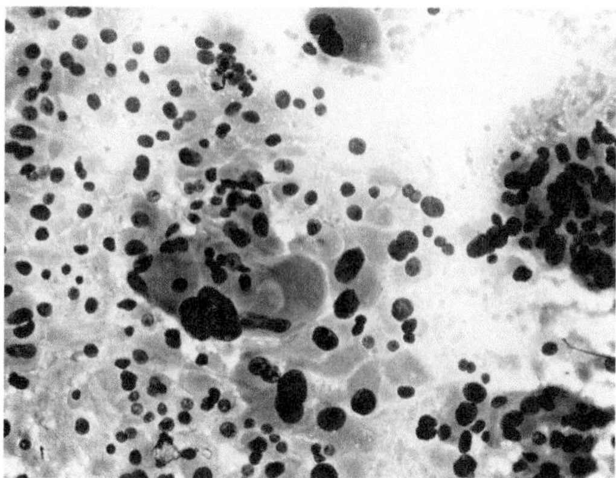

Fig. 10. Undifferentiated anaplastic thyroid carcinoma. Malignant cells with enlarged, irregular, pleomorphic nuclei, in clusters and discohesive, including giant multinucleated tumor cells (Diff-Quik ×40).

INDETERMINATE THYROID LESIONS

Considering the more nuanced diagnostic criteria, the management decisions, and the vast array of additional testing developed for indeterminate samples in the past few years, a more detailed description of the Bethesda III–V categories is beneficial. In the past, the "indeterminate" category has been a source of confusion for pathologists and clinicians and cases diagnosed as "atypical," follicular neoplasm," and "suspicious for malignancy" were lumped together in one category. Today, with the help of a significant armamentarium of molecular tests to rule in or rule out malignancy, more refined risk stratification exists for the indeterminate cases.

Atypia of Undetermined Significance/Follicular Lesion of Undetermined Significance

The Bethesda III category (AUS/FLUS) is a heterogeneous category in which the architectural and/or cytologic atypia is not sufficient to be classified as suspicious for follicular neoplasm, SFM, or malignant but is more than confidently diagnosed as benign.[4,5] Some of the common scenarios are (1) samples with a predominance of microfollicles in a hypocellular specimen with scant colloid (**Fig. 11**), (2) samples with a predominance of Hürthle cells in a hypocellular specimen with scant colloid, (3) focal features suggestive of papillary carcinoma (nuclear grooves, enlarged nuclei with pale chromatin, and alterations in nuclear contour) in an otherwise benign-appearing sample, (4) a minor population of follicular cells with nuclear enlargement and with prominent nucleoli in a patient with a history of radioactive iodine treatment, and (5) atypical cyst-lining cells with nuclear grooves and prominent nucleoli in an otherwise predominantly benign-appearing sample.[4] Given the heterogeneity of this category and the difficulty of providing specific criteria, encountering fair reproducibility among different pathologists and different institutions is expected. Clinicians should be aware that this is a category of last resort and pathologists make significant efforts not to use this designation indiscriminately. The frequency of AUS/FLUS interpretation should be approximately 7% of all thyroid FNA interpretations.[4]

Most AUS cases are based on follicular cell atypia, but in rare circumstances, the AUS designation is used for nonfollicular and/or nonepithelial atypia, such as atypical lymphoid infiltrate in a setting of Hashimoto thyroiditis, concerning for a low-grade lymphoma.

If an aspirate is diagnosed as AUS, it is implied that the sample met the adequacy criteria. When the diagnosis line is AUS, most pathologists use comments to further

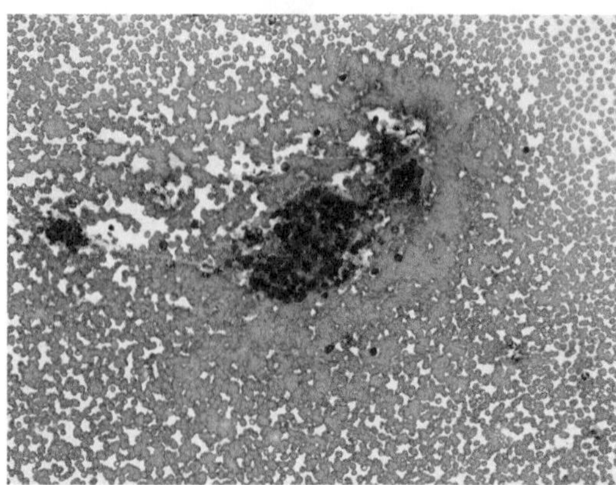

Fig. 11. AUS. Hypocellular specimen with rare groups of follicular cells in microfollicular architecture (Diff-Quik ×20).

describe the findings, list a differential diagnosis, and suggest follow-up recommendations, if applicable.

Example: FNA of a nodule in a patient with a history of Hashimoto thyroiditis. Sample is composed exclusively of Hürthle cells. Diagnosis: atypia of undetermined significance; specimen composed exclusively of Hürthle cells. Note: in a patient with a Hashimoto thyroiditis, the findings likely represent a Hürthle cell hyperplasia but a Hürthle cell neoplasm cannot be excluded. Clinical correlation is recommended.[4]

The recommended management for an initial AUS is the clinical correlation and a repeat FNA at 3 to 6 months or diagnostic thyroid surgery.

Follicular Neoplasm/Suspicious for Follicular Neoplasm

The Bethesda IV category (FN/SFN) is defined as a cellular aspirate composed of follicular cells with microfollicular architecture or demonstrating significant cell crowding. Colloid is usually scant or absent and some nuclear atypia (nuclear enlargement and prominent nucleoli) may be present. The hallmark of this category is the presence of an abnormal architecture (architectural atypia), usually in a highly cellular specimen (**Fig. 12**).

One important entity in the differential diagnosis in this category is parathyroid adenoma. A parathyroid adenoma may be misinterpreted as a "thyroid nodule" on ultrasound, and the sample submitted as "thyroid FNA" shows a crowded, highly cellular sample with cells resembling follicular cells. Immunohistochemical stains for parathormone and/or thyroglobulin identifies the cell of origin.

The diagnosis of FN/SFN is self-explanatory and an explicative note is optional.

The recommended management of a patient with FN/SFN is surgical excision. Because most patients undergo surgical excision (lobectomy or hemithyroidectomy), there are significant data in the literature regarding the positive predictive value of such a diagnosis. The likelihood of neoplasia is 65% to 85% and the risk of malignancy is 10% to 30%.[10]

Included in the same category is FN/SFN, Hürthle cell type (FNHTC/SFNHCT), which describes a sample composed predominantly of Hürthle cells demonstrating cellular and architectural atypia. Cellular atypia is manifested as nuclear enlargement, prominent nucleoli, high nucleus/cytoplasm ratio, or significant variability in nuclear size (at least 2×). Architectural atypia manifests as crowding and syncytial-like arrangement, although for Hürthle cell neoplasms, the cytologic atypia trumps

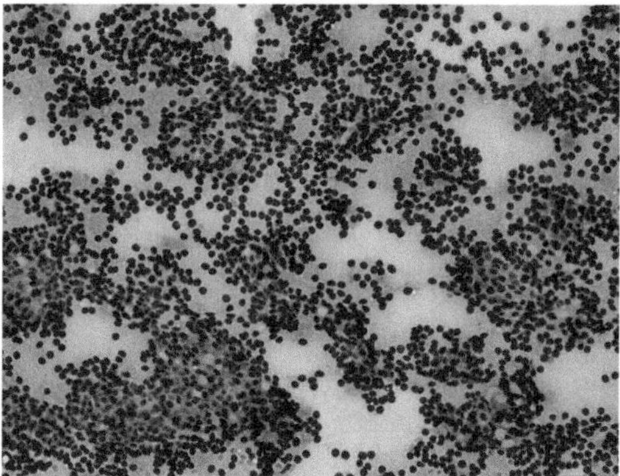

Fig. 12. Follicular neoplasm. Hypercellular specimen with follicular cells in microfollicular arrangements. Colloid is absent (Diff-Quik ×20).

architectural atypia. If a sample diagnosed as FN/SFN demonstrates only focal Hürthle cell differentiation, the World Heath Organization recommends that the designation FNHCT/SFNHTC should be used when at least 75% of the cells show Hürthle cell phenotype (**Figs. 13** and **14**).

The differential diagnosis of an FNHCT/SFNHCT includes Hürthle cell hyperplasia in a patient with lymphocytic thyroiditis and medullary carcinoma. In most patients with lymphocytic thyroiditis, a significant number of lymphocytes are present in the sample. There are cases of lymphocytic thyroiditis, however, in which the lymphoid component is absent or inconspicuous and the metaplastic Hürthle cells form nodules. In such cases, a Hürthle cell neoplasm cannot be excluded and both AUS with an explanatory note (discussed previously) and FNHCT/SFNHCT are acceptable diagnoses.

Some of the cytologic features of medullary thyroid carcinoma overlap with those of Hürthle cell neoplasms: granular cytoplasm; lack of colloid; and discohesive, isolated tumor cells. Unlike Hürthle cells, medullary carcinoma cells have inconspicuous nucleoli, some cells may show spindle cell features, and in many cases amyloid deposits are present on the slide. The diagnosis becomes easy when immunohistochemical stains for calcitonin and thyroglobulin are performed. Medullary carcinoma is positive for calcitonin and negative for thyroglobulin, whereas Hürthle cell neoplasms demonstrate the opposite pattern.

Bethesda V Category (Suspicious for Malignancy)

A specimen is SFM when some features of malignancy raise a strong suspicion for malignancy but the findings are not sufficient for a definitive diagnosis. Most primary thyroid malignancies have distinctive cytologic features, and a diagnosis of papillary carcinoma, medullary carcinoma, and lymphoma is usually straightforward. Exception from this rule is follicular carcinoma (included in category IV).

In some circumstances, however, the criteria for malignancy are not met, either qualitatively or quantitatively, for a variety of reasons, including uncommon variants of the respective malignancies, overlapping features with benign conditions (lymphocytic thyroiditis), and suboptimal sampling. Although in most cases papillary carcinoma is by far the one malignancy that may not display all cytologic features necessary for diagnosis, this category is heterogeneous and any malignancy, primary or metastatic, may be included.

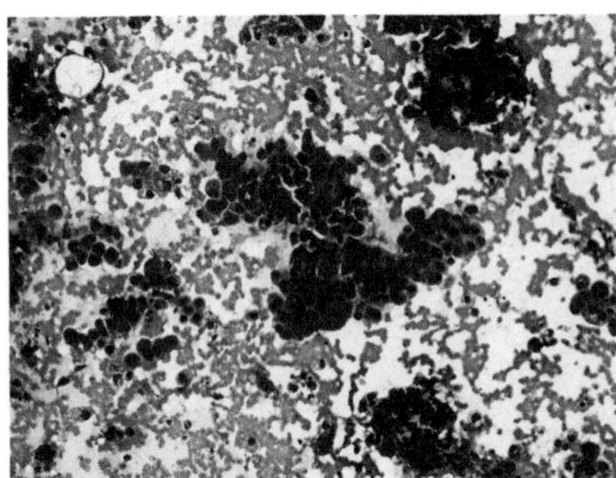

Fig. 13. Suspicious for follicular neoplasm Hürthle cell type. Cellular specimen with predominantly Hürthle cells, some colloid and few macrophages also present (Diff-Qick ×20).

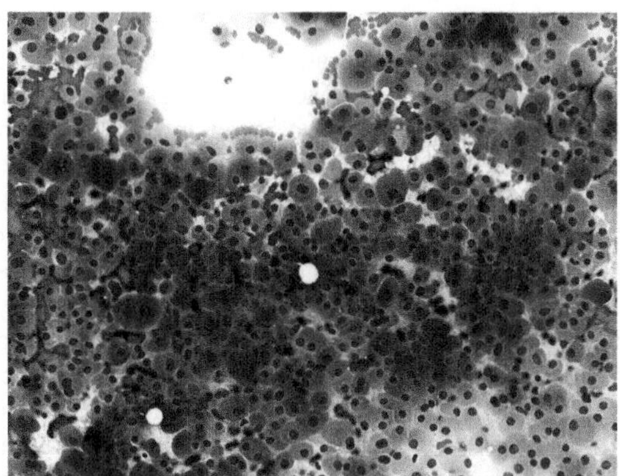

Fig. 14. Follicular neoplasm Hürthle cell type. Hypercellular specimen with only Hürthle cells. Colloid is absent (Diff-Quick ×20).

One of the most common scenarios is presence of either patchy or incomplete nuclear changes for papillary carcinoma. It means that the sample contains a minority of cells showing nuclear enlargement, nuclear pallor, nuclear grooves, and irregular nuclear contour but not nuclear inclusions, in a background of benign appearing follicular cells (**Fig. 15**), or a majority of the cells in the sample display only soft criteria of PTC (enlargement, clearing, and some nuclear membrane irregularity) but not grooves and inclusions. Another pattern is a sparsely cellular specimen in which many of the features of PTC (or medullary carcinoma, lymphoma) are present but the specimen is paucicellular.

The diagnosis, SFM, is an indication for surgery. The positive predictive value of this category is in the range of 60% to 75%[10] and in some studies up to 85%.

Ancillary Studies

Ancillary serologic studies, immunohistochemical stains and molecular tests are of great value in category IV and especially in category V and in many cases help patients and surgeons plan the extent of surgery and evaluate the advantage of performing intraoperative frozen section.

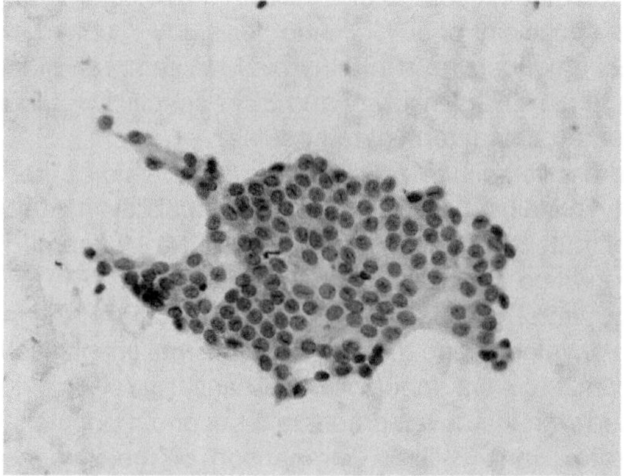

Fig. 15. Suspicious for papillary carcinoma. The picture is taken from a hypocellular specimen with few monolayers of follicular cells showing nuclear grooves but no inclusions. Other follicular groups show no atypia (PAP ×40).

Before the era of molecular testing, a vast majority of patients with thyroid nodules included in categories III, IV, and V were subjected to "diagnostic" surgery, with significant morbidity and health care costs. Moreover, a significant percentage of these patients who are diagnosed with thyroid carcinoma undergo a second surgical procedure, a completion thyroidectomy, which adds costs and morbidity.

The Bethesda System for Reporting Thyroid Cytology is a huge step forward in classification and diagnosis of thyroid nodules and comes with defined risks for malignancy for each of the 6 categories. Despite the major effort made by the National Cancer Institute panel involved in this project, it is accepted that cytology alone has limitations and does not provide a definitive diagnosis in one-third of the patients: those with indeterminate nodules. Without the aid of ancillary studies, the positive predictive value for malignancy in each of the indeterminate categories will not improve. This challenge led to significant scientific work to understand thyroid carcinogenesis and to develop immunohistochemical and molecular markers that will improve the specificity and sensitivity of FNA cytology.

Immunohistochemistry is widely used in all pathology laboratories; it does not require the specialized equipment or personnel of a molecular laboratory to perform and interpret the results, and, therefore, theoretically it represents an ideal assay for analysis of indeterminate thyroid nodules.[11] Unfortunately, numerous efforts to identify valuable markers with high specificity for carcinoma remained unsuccessful and it can be stated that in the last years the progress made in this field did not meet the expectations. Results can be improved by using the following immunohistochemistry markers in combination: galectin-3, HBME1, and cytokeratin-19 (CK19).

Galectin-3 is one of the most studied markers in thyroid neoplasia.[12] One of the largest studies[13] analyzing galectin-3 expression in indeterminate thyroid nodules found a sensitivity of 78%, specificity of 93%, and a negative predictive value of 91%. Because of a low sensitivity, galectin failed to establish itself as a stand-alone reliable marker of thyroid carcinoma.

HBME-1, which is antigen on the microvilli of mesothelioma cells, and CK19 that is part of the cytoskeleton of epithelial cells have been studied individually or in various combinations. CK19 had 76% sensitivity and 90% specificity at differentiating benign from malignant indeterminate lesions.[14] When a combination of CK19 and galectin-3 was used in oncocytic thyroid nodules only, specificity and sensitivity increased to 100%. The highest sensitivity and specificity in oncocytic and conventional thyroid samples were found when galectin-3 and HBME1 were combined, reaching a sensitivity of 97% and a specificity of 90%.[14] Another study[15] looked at a combination of HBME-1 and CK19 immunostains in 150 thyroid FNA samples, of which 48 were indeterminate, and found a 100% sensitivity and 85% specificity at identifying malignant nodules in the category of indeterminate nodules.

Despite the impressive results reported by these studies, technical difficulties, especially variability in staining and interobserver variability in interpretation of a stain performed on scant material of an FNA sample, limit the widespread adoption of these stains in the daily practice.

Over the past few years, a monoclonal antibody specific for the mutated BRAF protein (VE1) has been developed and tested in multiple malignancies that carry the BRAF V600E mutation, with excellent specificity and sensitivity.[16] The number of available antibodies increased with the development of a second monoclonal antibody against mutated BRAF protein (anti B-Raf). Comparison of the 2 monoclonal antibodies showed a concordance rate between immunohistochemistry and mutational analyses of 97% for VE1 and 88% for anti–B-Raf. Sensitivity and specificity were found to be 98% and 97% for VE1 and 95% and 83% for anti–B-Raf, respectively, indicating a better performance of VE1 compared with anti–B-Raf in an automated staining platform.[17]

Immunohistochemistry stain for BRAF V600E mutation is a promising alternative to molecular testing that is cheaper, faster, and easily available to smaller practices that are not equipped with a molecular laboratory. It can be successfully performed on an automated platform on cytology samples, cell blocks, and even smears. The presence of mutated BRAF protein plays multiple roles, because diagnostic and prognostic marker and may also have important implications in therapeutic decisions (less in differentiated thyroid cancer and more in other tumors carrying the V600E mutation). Unfortunately, despite the significant progress represented by the development of a monoclonal antibody specific for BRAF mutation with a positive predictive value close to 100%, only approximately 45% of PTC, classic type, and less than 10% of follicular variant of PTC (FVPTC) carry the BRAF V600E mutation.[18,19] The low prevalence of this mutation in FVPTC decreases the value of the antibody as a diagnostic tool in indeterminate FNA samples.

It is clear from this list of antibodies that each one of these markers has its own flaws and no marker proved to perfectly differentiate between indeterminate and malignant thyroid nodules.

In parallel to the development of immunomarkers, major progress has been made in the area of molecular testing.

Two major groups of molecular markers have shown promise as ancillary markers that increase diagnostic accuracy in real-life scenarios: somatic mutations (BRAF, RAS, RET/PTC, and PAX8/PPARγ mutations or translocations) and gene expression analysis (Afirma gene classifier [Veracyte, San Francisco, CA, USA]). MicroRNA (miRNA) expression analysis is currently used in research settings but it is expected to enter the mainstream of thyroid FNA testing in the future.

Molecular testing for BRAF V600E, the most common mutation in differentiated classic papillary carcinoma, has become widely available and many molecular laboratories offer BRAF mutation detection by polymerase chain reaction and sequencing on fresh FNA aspirates or formalin-fixed, paraffin-embedded samples.

Given the low prevalence of somatic mutations and translocations in thyroid carcinomas, and the mutually exclusive nature of them,[19] none of them is used as a stand-alone test to differentiate benign from malignant indeterminate FNA. They are used in various panels commercially available or developed and performed by selected molecular laboratories. FDA has recently approved the miR*Inform* panel (Asuragen, Austin, TX, USA) to be used as a diagnostic tool in indeterminate nodules. Recent studies in the literature put the sensitivity of this panel approximately 92%, making a compelling argument that patients who have a positive mutation panel should undergo a total thyroidectomy as the initial surgery.[20,21]

Developed as a rule-out carcinoma test, the Veracyte Afirma gene classifier is a multigene expression classifier that uses a proprietary algorithm to distinguish benign from suspicious thyroid nodules. On large sample studies, the Veracyte test demonstrated a specificity of 52% and a negative predictive value of 95% for Bethesda III, 94% for Bethesda IV, and 85% for Bethesda V categories.[22]

Because approximately half of the indeterminate nodules demonstrate a benign gene profile, this test leads to a significant reduction of unnecessary surgeries in indeterminate nodules.

The indications and the sequence in which all these molecular tests are used in daily practice varies from one institution to another and in many hospitals diagnostic algorithms are developed as a collaborative effort between pathology, endocrinology, and surgery departments.

In conclusion, more scientific progress is expected to occur in the field of thyroid carcinogenesis and in the ability to differentiate indeterminate from malignant nodules. The next-generation sequencing is the newest addition to the molecular testing. Currently, several panels are being developed, using cytology material from FNAs, with multiple gene mutations and gene fusions promising to be of diagnostic and prognostic importance. There is also a large body of work currently in the field of miRNA expression in a variety of malignancies, and hopefully development of miRNA panels run on FNA samples will bring a solution to the diagnostic difficulties encountered today, a solution that is not only viable but also cost effective.

REFERENCES

1. Barnes L. Surgical pathology of the head and neck. In: Barnes L, editor. 3rd edition. Zug (Switzerland): Informa Healthcare; 2009. p. 1–20.
2. Cibas ES, Ali SZ. The Bethesda system for reporting thyroid cytopathology. Am J Clin Pathol 2009;132(5):658–65.
3. Lewis CM, Chang K. Thyroid fine-needle aspiration biopsy: variability in reporting. Thyroid 2009;19(7):717–23.
4. Syed Z, Ali ES, editors. The Bethesda system for reporting thyroid cytopathology. Definitions, criteria and explanatory notes. Newyork: Springer; 2010.
5. Baloch ZW, LiVolsi VA, Asa SL, et al. Diagnostic terminology and morphologic criteria for cytologic diagnosis of thyroid lesions: a synopsis of the National Cancer Insitute Thyroid Fine-Needle Aspiration State of the Science Conference. Diagn Cytopathol 2008;36(6):425–37.
6. Kiri SR. Thyroid cytopathology: atlas and text. Philadelphia: Lippincott Williams & Wilkins; 2008.
7. Volante M, Landolfi S, Chiusa L, et al. Poorly differentiated carcinoma of the thyroid with trabecular, insular and solid paterns: a clinicopathologic study od 183 patients. Cancer 2004;100(5):950–7.
8. Kossev P, Livolsi V. Lymphoid lesions of the thyroid: review in light of the revised Europian American Lymphoma classification and upcoming WHO classification. Thyroid 1999;9(12):1273–80.
9. Ivy HK. Cancer metastatic to the thyroid: a diagnostic problem. Mayo Clin Proc 1984;59(12):856–9.
10. Cooper DS, Doherty GM, Haugen BR, et al. Management guidelines for patients with thyroid nodules and differentiated thyroid cancer. Thyroid 2006;16(2):109–42.
11. Griffith OL, Chiu CG, Gown AM, et al. Biomarker panel diagnosis of thyroid cancer: a critical review. Expert Rev Anticancer Ther 2008;8(9):1399–413.
12. Chiu CG, Strugnell SS, Griffith OL, et al. Diagnostic utility of galectin-3 in thyroid cancer. Am J Pathol 2010;176(5):2067–81.
13. Bartolazzi A, Orlandi F, Saggiorato E, et al. Galectin-3-expression analysis in the surgical selection of follicular thyroid nodules with indeterminate fine-needle aspiration cytology: a prospective multicentre study. Lancet Oncol 2008;9(6):543–9.
14. Saggiorato E, De Pompa R, Volante M, et al. Characterization of thyroid "follicular neoplasms" in fine-needle aspiration cytological specimens using a panel of immunohistochemical markers: a proposal for clinical application. Endocr Relat Cancer 2005;12(2):305–17.
15. Cochand-Priollet B, Dahan H, Laloi-Michelin M, et al. Immunocytochemistry with cytokeratin 19 and anti-human mesothelial cell antibody (HBME1) increases the diagnostic accuracy of thyroid fine-needle aspirations: preliminary report of 150

liquid-based fine-needle aspirations with histological control. Thyroid 2011; 21(10):1067–73.
16. Koperek O, Kornauth C, Capper D, et al. Immunohistochemical detection of the BRAF V600E-mutated protein in papillary thyroid carcinoma. Am J Surg Pathol 2012;36(6):844–50.
17. Routhier CA, Mochel MC, Lynch K, et al. Comparison of 2 monoclonal antibodies for immunohistochemical detection of BRAF V600E mutation in malignant melanoma, pulmonary carcinoma, gastrointestinal carcinoma, thyroid carcinoma, and gliomas. Hum Pathol 2013;44(11):2563–70.
18. Nikiforov YE. Thyroid carcinoma: molecular pathways and therapeutic targets. Mod Pathol 2008;21(Suppl 2):S37–43.
19. Nikiforov YE. Molecular analysis of thyroid tumors. Mod Pathol 2011;24(Suppl 2): S34–43.
20. Nikiforov YE, Ohori NP, Hodak SP, et al. Impact of mutational testing on the diagnosis and management of patients with cytologically indeterminate thyroid nodules: a prospective analysis of 1056 FNA samples. J Clin Endocrinol Metab 2011;96(11):3390–7.
21. Filicori F, Keutgen XM, Buitrago D, et al. Risk stratification of indeterminate thyroid fine-needle aspiration biopsy specimens based on mutation analysis. Surgery 2011;150(6):1085–91.
22. Alexander EK, Kennedy GC, Baloch ZW, et al. Preoperative diagnosis of benign thyroid nodules with indeterminate cytology. N Engl J Med 2012;367(8):705–15.

Clinician-Performed Thyroid Ultrasound

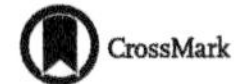

Marc D. Coltrera, MD[a,b,*]

KEYWORDS

• Ultrasound • Office-based • Thyroid cancer • Training • Validation • Competency

KEY POINTS

- Thyroid ultrasounds require initial training, validation, and establishment of competency.
- When selecting a clinic-based ultrasound, one should consider the important features and capabilities.
- The economics of an ultrasound purchase come down to what is achievable when it comes to medical billing.
- There are important ultrasound findings associated with thyroid malignancy.
- There is unparalleled usefulness for ultrasound in the operating room just before the incision.

INTRODUCTION

The role of ultrasound is widely acknowledged by radiology experts as the primary imaging modality for diseases of the thyroid. As its use has expanded and the technology has improved placing less-expensive, higher-resolution machines in the hands of nonradiologists, ultrasound has also created an important role for itself in the routine examination of cervical lymph nodes and head and neck masses outside of the central compartment. In the past decade, much has been written and much effort has been expended to increase the routine clinical use of ultrasound by head and neck surgeons. Beyond the initial diagnosis, the usefulness of ultrasound for surgical planning just before incision is unparalleled.

Disclosure Statement: The author has no actual or potential conflict of interest, including employment, consultancies, stock ownership, patent applications/registrations, grants, and other funding.

[a] Department of OTO-HNS, University of Washington, 1959 Northeast Pacific, Box 356515, Seattle, WA 98195, USA; [b] OTO-HNS Division, VA Puget Sound, 1660 S Columbian Way, Seattle, WA 98108, USA

* Department of OTO-HNS, University of Washington, 1959 Northeast Pacific, Box 356515, Seattle, WA 98195.

E-mail address: Coltrera@u.washington.edu

Otolaryngol Clin N Am 47 (2014) 491–507
http://dx.doi.org/10.1016/j.otc.2014.04.001 oto.theclinics.com
0030-6665/14/$ – see front matter

This article is not written to convince the reader that they should seek training in ultrasound, but it is intended to demystify the process for those with a potential interest. It does not aim to cover ultrasound findings in depth. Instead, it is focused on the bare minimum requirements and considerations involved in clinician-performed ultrasound. Further readings are listed at the end of the article to direct the reader to some excellent texts to help build confidence and experience. The topic of ultrasound-guided fine-needle aspiration (FNA) is addressed separately in another article by Orloff and colleagues in this issue.

INITIAL ULTRASOUND TRAINING

At the current time in the United States, training of nonradiologist specialists in ultrasound presents a bit of a conundrum. It has been an integrated part of obstetrics and gynecology residency programs for well more than a decade. More recently, the use of ultrasound in trauma evaluations, such as the Focused Assessment with Sonography for Trauma examination, has been part of formalized residency training for general surgeons and emergency medical specialists. For most specialists, notably otolaryngologists interested in general neck examination applications and others interested in endocrine applications specifically, the formal training has been much more limited. Sponsored training programs in the United States have been primarily in the form of introductory postgraduate courses.

With respect to thyroid and parathyroid applications, there are now 3 organizations within the United States offering postgraduate training programs: the American Association of Clinical Endocrinologists (AACE, www.aace.org), the American College of Surgeons (www.facs.org), and the American Academy of Otolaryngology-Head and Neck Surgery (AAO-HNS, www.entnet.org). These organizations offer 1- and 2-day postgraduate courses aimed at introducing the practicing clinician to the basics of ultrasound. The courses include a precourse preparation package and at least a half day of didactics covering ultrasound physics, basic instrumentation (also known as knobology), basic image interpretation, and clinical applications (for an example, see Ref.[1]). The second half of a 1-day course is spent in a hands-on practice session. The culmination of the course is a practical examination and the awarding of a certificate from the sponsoring group.

The practical issue remains as follows: What does a 1- or 2-day course actually prepare the clinician for? At best, these courses are a cursory introduction to ultrasound techniques; this single fact has led to a general discounting of their worth by medical insurers among others and used as a justification to deny payment for services such as image-guided FNA. It is generally agreed that the best way to train nonradiologist clinicians in ultrasound techniques is by integrating the training into the respective residency training programs (eg, the American Board of Otolaryngology, www.aboto.org). Efforts to do so are currently ongoing, but such an approach clearly leaves out most of the practicing specialty clinicians for the next decade or so unless there is a mechanism to fully train and assess competency among clinicians within a postgraduate setting.

OBTAINING ADEQUATE EXPERIENCE: VALIDATION AND ASSESSMENT OF COMPETENCY

At the present time, there is no formal validation process for head and neck surgeons to further their ultrasound training beyond the initial course, though there are active initiatives to institute one.[1] Through the auspices of the AACE, endocrinologists have been several years ahead of head and neck surgeons in actively supporting postgraduate ultrasound education. A relationship between the AACE and the American

Institute for Ultrasound Medicine (AIUM, www.aium.org) has led to the creation of a voluntary peer-review process, the AIUM Ultrasound Practice Accreditation program. This program includes a formal mechanism for submitting cases for review leading to initial accreditation and includes a requirement for reaccreditation every 3 years. This type of program meets the requirements of many insurance organizations and holds the promise of increased standardization leading to better outcomes.

At the conclusion of the 1- and 2-day courses, attendees are instructed to seek a mentorship with an experienced colleague, a radiologist, or radiology department performing head and neck ultrasound. Ongoing self-evaluation and feedback can be an important part of continuously honing skills and as part of a recurrent training process. An example of this is an almost-daily exercise the author avails himself of in his clinical practice. When performing a focused portable ultrasound examination in the clinic as part of a full head and neck examination in preparation for a FNA, the portable examination findings are compared with the more complete formal ultrasound examination obtained in the radiology department's ultrasound suite. The reader should rightly ask the following: How confident can the neophyte nonradiologist ultrasonographer be in this type of training process, and how much experience is necessary to obtain a satisfactory level of competence?

Defining competency is one of the central issues in all of medical education. Residency education within the United States has recently been completely reengineered around the assessment of core competencies.[2] Under the older system, surgically oriented resident educational progress was assessed principally by the number of procedures performed as an assistant and as a primary surgeon. Under the new system, the number of procedures is still tracked, but the emphasis is placed on the continuous evaluation of a set of skills. For nonradiologist specialty ultrasound training, self-assessment with the help of a mentor is the currently touted mechanism. Seen from the vantage point of core competencies, is this a viable training methodology, and can adequate competency be achieved under these conditions?

To help answer the questions, it is instructive to look at the current training for sonographers and radiology residents (sonologists) in the United States and Canada as a point of comparison. Sonographers are the technicians who perform most of the ultrasound examinations. The American Institute for Ultrasound in Medicine (AIUM, www.aium.org) publishes the accreditation standards in the United States, and the Canadian Society of Diagnostic Medical Sonographers (www.csdms.org) publishes them in Canada. When it comes to actually performing the ultrasound examinations, their training is the most extensive and includes 300 to 500 procedures performed over a 2- to 3-year period. In contrast, radiologists, accredited by the American College of Radiology (www.acr.org) in the United States and by the Royal College of Physicians and Surgeons of Canada (www.royalcollege.ca), spend approximately 6 months of their residencies in dedicated ultrasound interpretation training.

These gold standards of training are extensive and comprehensive; but when broken down into the different body areas, the time spent on any single area, such as the head and neck region, is much more approachable for nonradiologist specialists. Obstetrics and gynecology ultrasound is arguably the largest ultrasound segment in radiology residencies. Seventy-five percent of radiology residents spend less than 4 weeks per year over a 2-year period obtaining experience in this area.[3] What is particularly interesting is that 30% of their experience is obtained outside of the radiology department and 40% is estimated to occur after hours without an attending present at the time of the examination. In effect, much of the ultrasound training occurs through examination comparison with a mentor, which is precisely the same situation that nonradiologist specialists are faced with when seeking validation and assessment of competency.

As for the issue of how many examinations are required to achieve an acceptable level of competency, several studies of the learning curve in ultrasound examination have established that an average of 25 to 50 focused examinations are needed to achieve greater than 90% concordance with a radiologist's interpretation of the same examination.[4–6] A recent article addressed the specific issue of observer experience (<2 years or >7 years) and evaluation of thyroid malignancy and lymph node metastases in 1421 patients.[7] Preoperative staging included extrathyroidal extension and ultrasound features of lymph node metastases, including shape, echogenicity, microcalcifications, cystic change, and vascularity. The two groups differed only in their ability to assess lateral neck compartment lymph node involvement (38.5% predictive for the <2-year group compared with 64% in the >7-year group).

Comparisons with radiologists may not answer all questions when it comes to competence. Studies have raised issues regarding the level of training for radiology residents and whether it is adequate in ultrasound.[8] The reasons for the lack of competence among radiologists present an interesting counterpart to the discussion of nonradiologist competence. One of the main problems for the radiologists in the study was the lack of detailed anatomic knowledge and the inability of 44% to identify anatomic landmarks. Considering the detailed anatomic knowledge of the head and neck region possessed by the average head and neck surgeon and the attainment of comparative competency in the focused ultrasound examination studies, an outside observer could easily conclude that achievement of competence in head and neck ultrasounds is well within the means of the average head and neck surgeon.

ESSENTIAL EQUIPMENT AND THE ECONOMICS OF CLINIC-BASED ULTRASOUND

The past 5 years has seen a substantial change in the ultrasound marketplace and the pricing of portable ultrasound units. Major companies envisioned the original market for ultrasound as being limited to the radiologic suite.[9] The significant increase in ultrasound-trained nonradiologist specialists has created a burgeoning market for more portable ultrasound units for use in obstetrics-gynecology, urology, otolaryngology, general surgery, orthopedics, neurosurgery, cardiology, vascular surgery, and emergency medicine, among others. The analytic electronics contained in the portable units are largely equivalent to those found in the larger radiologic suite units. The main differences are found in storage capacity, probe capability, and postimaging analysis.

Portable units are available from many manufacturers along with optional equipment, such as dedicated carts that can contribute substantially to the cost. **Fig. 1** is a real-world photograph of a unit the author uses routinely in an otolaryngology clinic setting. The essential elements are all evident in the photograph: a generic clinic cart with a drawer, a portable ultrasound unit, one linear multifrequency probe used for small-parts examinations, probe gel, saran wrap, and rubber bands (located in the drawer) for protecting the probe from blood during FNA. Units with more capability than the one in the picture are widely available for approximately $20,000 at the time of this writing.

Picking an ultrasound is a personal decision, and the reader is to be encouraged to try different units before purchasing. That being said, the ergonomics of the most common units are comparable and allow for increasingly easy transitions between units available throughout a hospital. There are literally hundreds of specifications and options listed in ultrasound brochures. The basic capabilities of a useful unit for head and neck examinations should include the following:

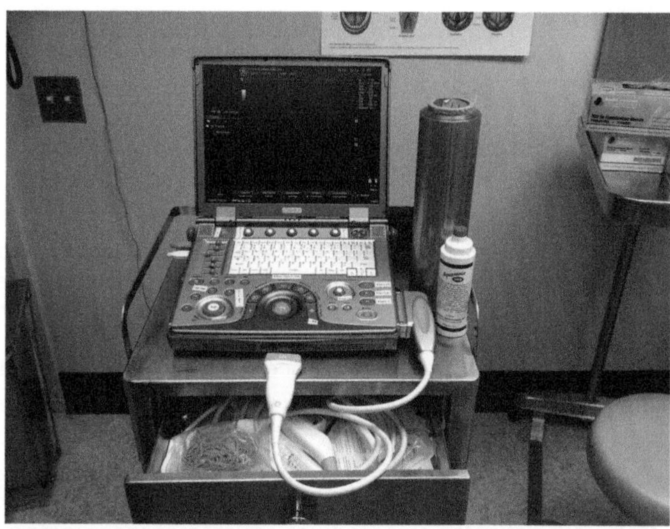

Fig. 1. Example of a real-world portable ultrasound unit used in the clinic setting. The basic items include a generic cart, the basic ultrasound unit, one multifrequency small-parts probe, and a recording device (eg, printer or DVD recorder on a lower shelf not seen in the photograph). See text for further details.

Monitor

High-resolution color LCD, diagonal dimension: 15 in, resolution: 1024 × 768.

Imaging Modes

B, color Doppler, power Doppler, duplex mode for B/Doppler, spatial compounding imaging for linear probes (desirable).

Cineloop Capabilities

Support for B, color Doppler, and power Doppler. The potential length/time of a cineloop depends on the maximum frame storage (>1000 frames is desirable) as well as the frame rate (see later discussion).

Transducer

A single, linear array, multifrequency probe for small parts. The most useful range of frequencies is 7.5 to 12.5 MHz for neck structures. Higher-frequency small-parts probes up to 15 MHz are becoming increasingly available and affordable. There are theoretical advantages to the higher frequencies when it comes to parathyroid localization. (See "Further readings" for more details and a discussion of ultrasound physics.)

Output Modalities

USB, Ethernet, S-video/VGA/composite video (can be achievable through USB adapters).

Peripherals

USB-connected storage unit and/or DVD recorder, programmable pedal footswitch (desirable) (The use of a footswitch can make FNA image capture significantly easier.)

Display Dynamic Range

100 dB (B mode).

Frame Rate

Approximately greater than 350 frames per second (varies with transducer in use as well as processing capabilities).

Bottom line on technical specifications

Additional technical specifications, such as processor speed, memory, and storage, all affect the capabilities of the unit; but beyond the basic specifications listed earlier, the comparison of individual technical specifications does not necessarily add significantly to the process of selecting a machine. Many times, it is easier to compare the general capabilities and the user experiences as surrogates for the underlying electronics.

Image documentation for medical billing

Image documentation is frequently necessary for the medical record and is required for medical billing purposes (see article by Orloff and colleagues in this issue). A programmable footswitch makes the process much easier for image recording as well as for unit adjustment during examinations performed by a solo clinician. The economics of an ultrasound purchase comes down to what is achievable when it comes to medical billing. In 2013, billing for clinical ultrasound in the United States involves 2 Current Procedural Terminology (CPT) code groups: 76536 and 76942/10022 (**Table 1**). The diagnostic code 76536 poses the greatest difficulty for the nonradiologist to achieve reimbursement with for understandable reasons. More rigorous proof of validation and competency through formalized accreditation mechanisms as mentioned earlier (eg, AIUM Ultrasound Practice Accreditation) should go a long way to easing this situation for the physician with postgraduate training. The incorporation of formal ultrasound training into residencies, such as obstetrics and gynecology, led to the recognition of ultrasound being part of the specialty's area of competence.

As the number of head and neck specialists trained in ultrasound continues to increase in both the postgraduate and residency arenas, medical reimbursement is also expected to become less of an issue. At the time of this writing, the most consistent results in achieving reimbursement have been seen in the technical area of FNA under ultrasound guidance using 76942/10022. Third-party payers frequently require some sort of petition from the nonradiologist care provider and documentation of formal training and mentorship. In at least one instance known to the author, the

Table 1
2013 Medicare physician fee schedule (averages)

CPT Code	Description	Global Payment ($)	Professional Payment ($)	Technical Payment ($)
76536	Diagnostic ultrasound of the soft tissues of the head and neck	124.86	27.22	97.65
76942	Ultrasound guidance for needle placement, imaging supervision, and interpretation	208.56	32.66	175.90
		Nonfacility Payment ($)		
10022	FNA with image guidance	141.20	—	—

petition and the documentation took the form of submitting multiple cases for reimbursement, which were then taken as proof of a consistent practice pattern. Barriers still remain to the incorporation of ultrasound into standard head and neck clinical practice. However, there is an increasing appreciation for the proper ways to accomplish it; the reader is referred to additional literature on the subject, including the demonstrated cost-effective nature of clinic-based ultrasound.[10,11]

THE ESSENTIAL ULTRASOUND FINDINGS

A comprehensive discussion of thyroid ultrasound findings as well as more general head and neck ultrasound findings is well beyond the scope of this article. The reader is referred to 3 excellent books on the subject listed at the end of the article. As previously stated, the focus of this article is to strip the subject of clinic-based ultrasound down to its essential elements; the evaluation of thyroid nodules essentially focuses on defining the risk of thyroid cancer.

Thyroid nodules occur in more than 50% of the general population, increasing with age, whereas palpable thyroid nodules (typically >1.5 cm in size) occur in only 5% to 8%.[12] What is even more pertinent to the subject at hand is the fact that up to 35% of thyroids examined at autopsy and surgery have the incidental finding of subcentimeter papillary carcinomas.[13,14] Whether efforts should be expended to diagnose let alone treat subcentimeter disease is a complex, evolving topic.[15] The problem for the nonradiologist clinician performing ultrasound is to understand the basic ultrasound findings that might direct FNA or lead to a decision to perform surgery for definitive diagnosis.

There are 7 ultrasound findings that are generally evaluated when considering nodules deemed suspicious enough to recommend FNA. Their relative importance varies when comparing published sonographic criteria sets. The general findings include:

1) Hypoechogenicity
2) Irregular (microlobulated) margins
3) Microcalcifications
4) Anteroposterior to transverse diameter ratio greater than 1 (eg, "taller than wide on transverse view")
5) Intranodular vascularity
6) Size
7) Significant growth.

Examples of the first 6 findings are demonstrated in **Figs. 2** and **3**.

There are 3 criteria sets (eg, guidelines) in wide use: the AACE,[16] the Kim criteria[17] and the Society of Radiologists in Ultrasound (SRU).[18]

- The **AACE's criteria** focus on hypoechoic nodules with one or more additional suspicious features. Size and significant growth are not emphasized.
- The **Kim criteria** include any single suspicious sonographic finding excluding size and vascularity.
- The **SRU's criteria** are stratified by size. Reading the consensus statement along with additional commentary, one of the reasons why the SRU's criteria included size was to acknowledge the data regarding a lack of clinical impact associated with subcentimeter nodules.[19] The SRU's criteria recommend biopsy for nodules that are 1.0 cm or greater with microcalcifications, nodules that are 1.5 cm or greater if solid or coarsely calcified, and nodules that are 2.0 cm or greater if mixed cystic and solid. The SRU's criteria also include the finding of significant

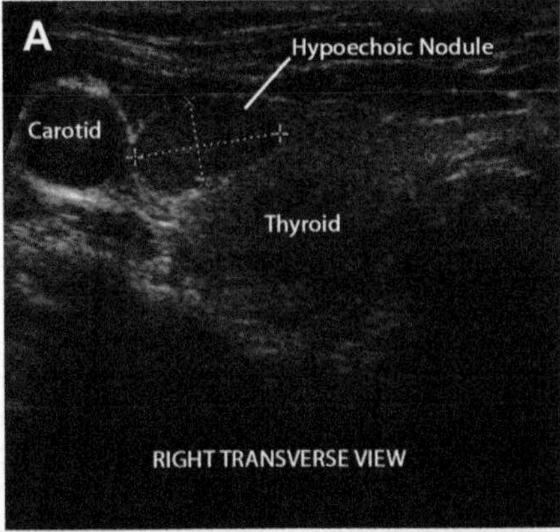

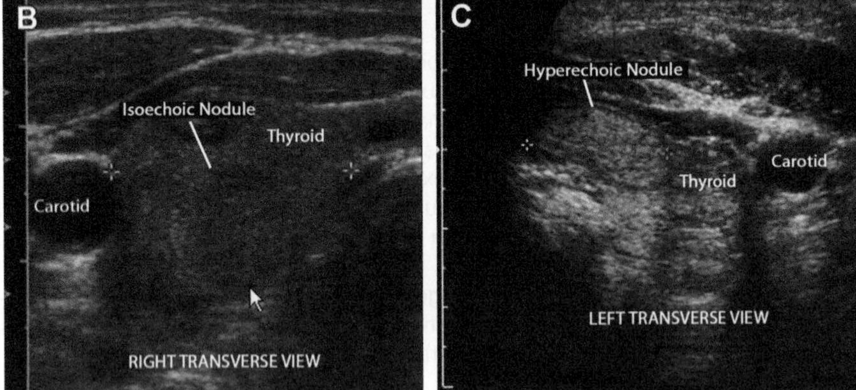

Fig. 2. Examples of (*A*) hypoechoic, (*B*) isoechoic, and (*C*) hyperechoic thyroid nodules. Nodule echogenicity is expressed relative to the adjacent thyroid tissue.

growth, but there is no clear definition of this. In general, it seems to be when the volume change over 6 months exceeds a 20% increase.

Comparison of the different criteria is complicated, and there are several articles that compare the different published guidelines favoring one or the other for different reasons.[20,21] In its simplest form, the most common sonographic findings associated with papillary thyroid carcinoma are hypoechogenicity (86%), microcalcifications (42%), and internal hypervascularity (69%).[22] In contrast, most follicular carcinomas are isoechoic or hyperechoic and lack calcifications. Sensitivity and specificity have to be considered when trying to make an informed judgment with regard to ultrasound findings, and clearly no single ultrasound finding is sufficient to make a diagnosis of malignancy (**Table 2**).[23–27] Although general sensitivity and specificity are low for the individual ultrasound criteria, the reader should recognize the importance of the overall result obtained by using ultrasound to select nodules for FNA cytologic analysis. Comparing high-risk nodules to low-risk nodules, the combined methods result in the ability to identify the 11% of patients with a 34% risk of malignancy and the 81% of patients with less than a 3% risk of malignancy.[28] Summing it up, the clinician should choose one of the more common guidelines, such as those mentioned earlier, and consistently apply the guideline criteria in their FNA decision-making process.

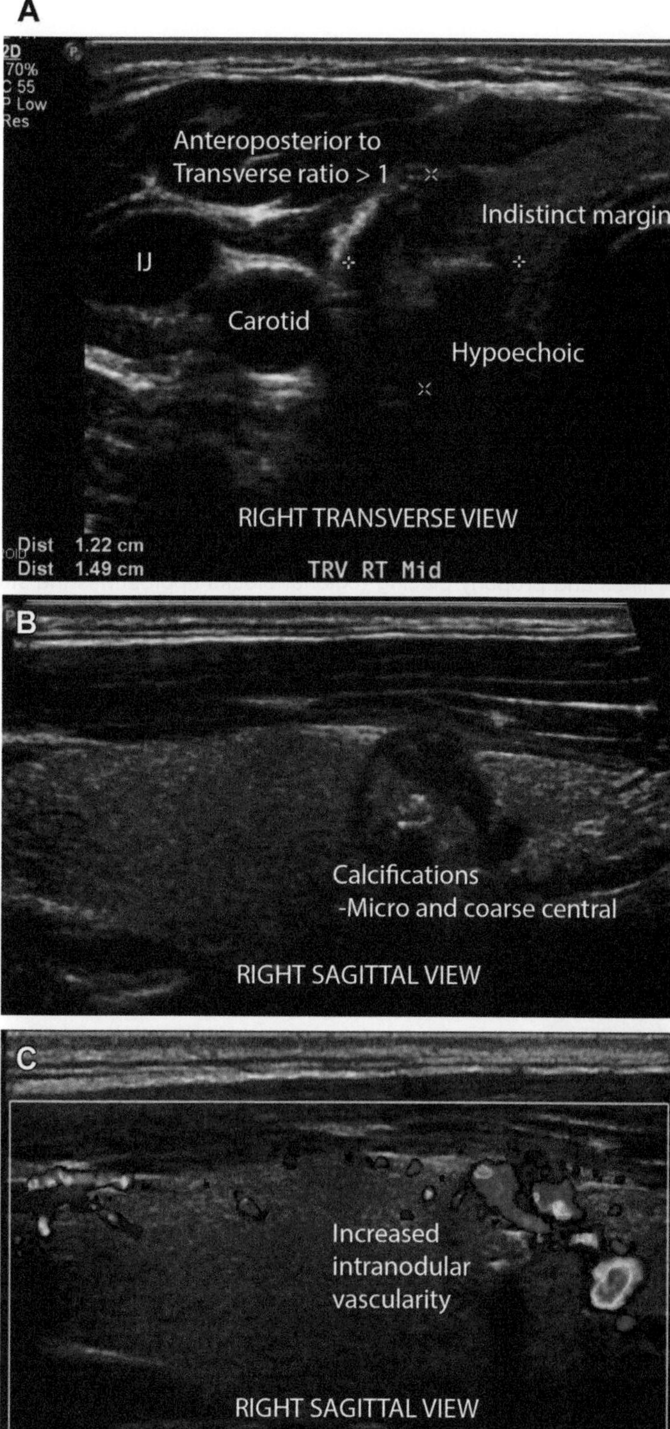

Fig. 3. Example of a thyroid nodule exhibiting all of the general ultrasound findings indicating need for FNA (*A–C*). The general findings include hypoechogenicity, irregular (microlobulated) margins, anteroposterior to transverse diameter ratio greater than 1, microcalcifications or course central calcifications, intranodular vascularity, and size of 1 cm or greater.

Table 2
Sensitivity and specificity of single ultrasound criteria (averages)

	Sensitivity (%)	Specificity (%)
Anteroposterior/transverse >1	40	90
Hypoechoic	80	53
Intranodular blood flow	67	81
Irregular margins	51	76
Loss of halo	66	43
Microcalcifications	43	90

USE OF ULTRASOUND IN THE OPERATING ROOM IN THE IMMEDIATE PREOPERATIVE SETTING

A random walk into most operating rooms in the United States will result in finding readily accessible portable ultrasound units (**Fig. 4**). The use of ultrasound for starting intravascular lines and properly placing regional blocks approaches the standard of care among anesthesiologists. These units are frequently available to other clinicians within the operating room suite. For the operative surgeon, ultrasound has a significant role to play in the operating room. The most common uses of true intraoperative ultrasound techniques are found in vascular surgery and abdominal procedures. The actual intraoperative use of ultrasound in the head and neck is very limited. The important role in the head and neck region is in the immediate preincision setting when patients are positioned on the table.

Ultrasound in Thyroid Surgery

In thyroid surgery, emphasis has been placed on performing surgeries through minimal-size incisions with a low neck placement for the best cosmetic effect. The

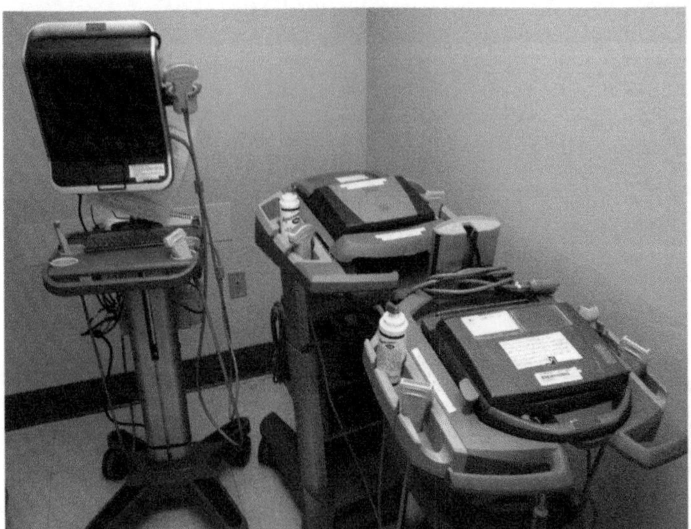

Fig. 4. A random walk into an anesthesia supply closet at a major hospital in the Northwest with 3 ultrasound units available for immediate preoperative incision planning.

worst-case scenario for many thyroid surgeons is a young woman with a long, thin neck. Techniques such as endoscopic procedures popularized by Miccoli and colleagues[29] have helped to improve cosmetics in select cases; but because of patient issues, equipment availability, and/or surgeon experience, a variation of the traditional open procedures still prevails in most cases. Localization of the thyroid using ultrasound after patients are positioned can help tremendously in designing minimal incisions and anticipating technical issues during the operation. The extent of the superior and inferior poles can be checked with respect to palpable landmarks, including the hyoid bone, cricoid and thyroid cartilages, and the clavicles (**Fig. 5**). The efficacy of neck extension can be evaluated objectively, and the degree of extension can be

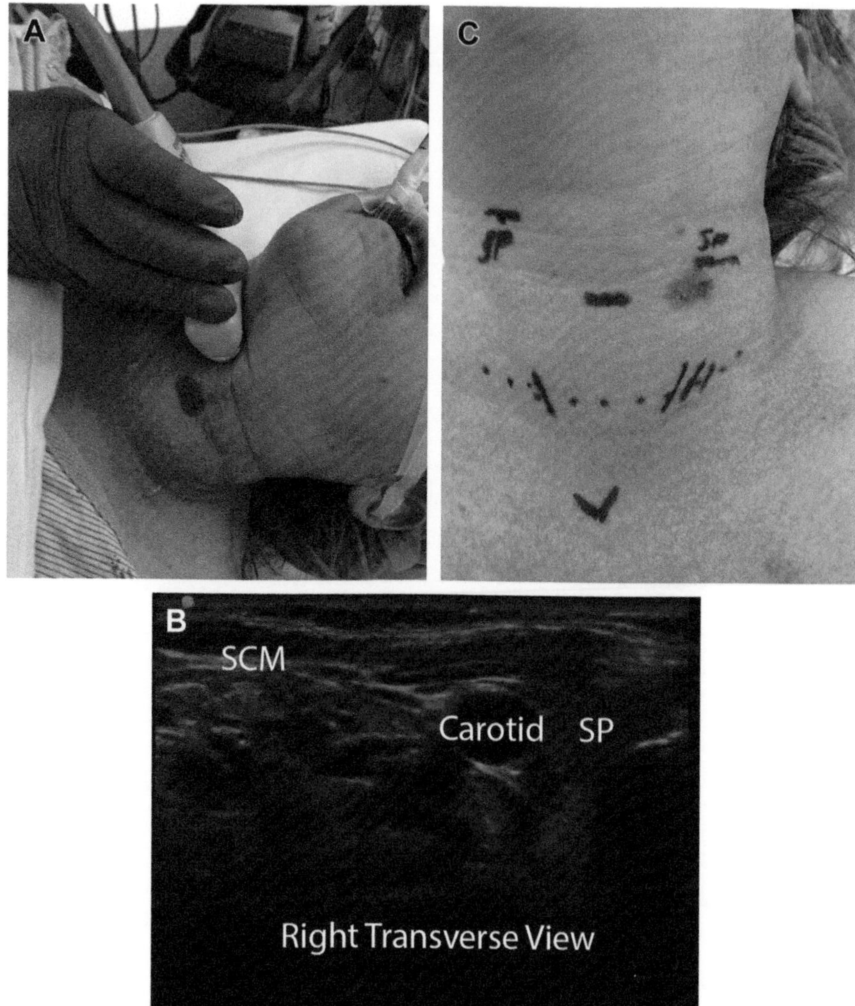

Fig. 5. (*A*) Immediate preincision ultrasound after patient is intubated and positioned. (*B*) Right transverse view following the thyroid superior pole (SP) at a point just above cricoid level. (*C*) The superior extent of the SP was marked along with other landmarks in an enlarged multinodular goiter case allowing for design of a minimal incision (4 cm) using standard surgical techniques. SCM, sternocleidomastoid muscle.

modified based on the change in position of the inferior and superior thyroid poles. Many times, neck extension does not help improve access to the thyroid and serves to elongate the superior extent of the gland, which can be counterproductive.

Pre-incision Ultrasound

In analogous fashion, preincision ultrasound can be useful to help locate the best position for a parathyroid exploration incision. Routine use of ultrasound after patients are positioned on the operating table also results in a somewhat surprising finding regarding the parathyroids: they are frequently mobile and can change their position significantly as the neck is manipulated. **Fig. 6** demonstrates a case with a large change in position based on alternating cricoid pressure and cricoid retraction. The

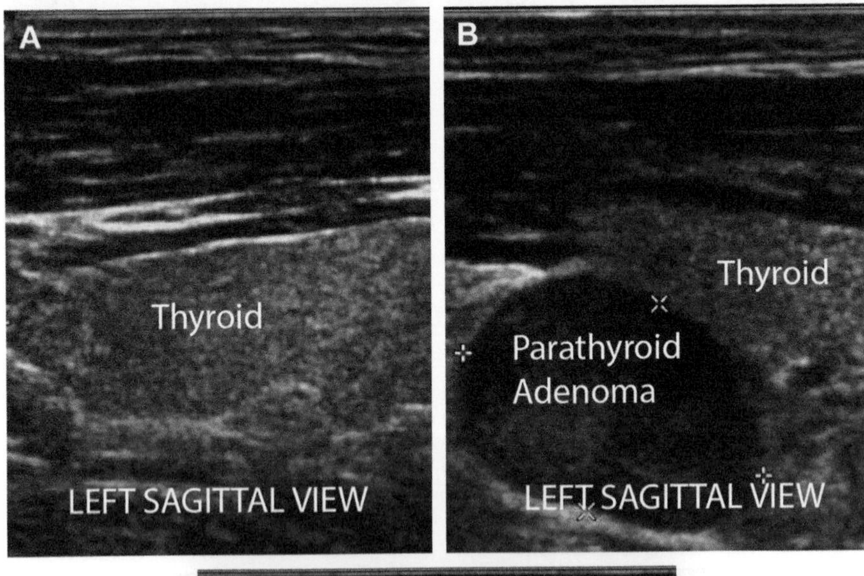

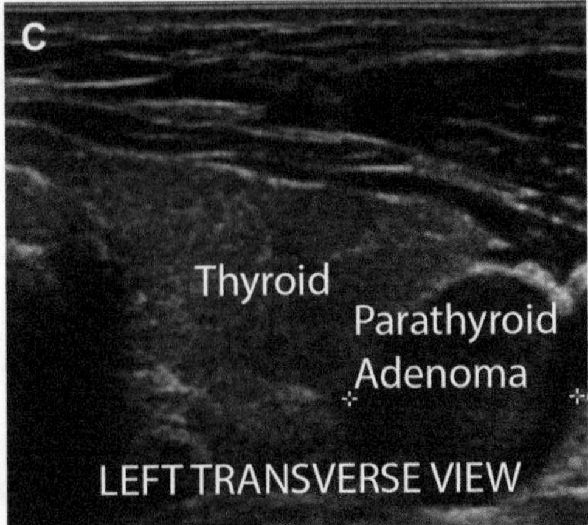

Fig. 6. (*A*) Left sagittal view of superior pole of thyroid without cricoid and tracheal pressure. (*B*) Left sagittal view of superior pole of the thyroid with cricoid and tracheal pressure demonstrating lateralization of a hypoechoic mass consistent with a parathyroid adenoma. (*C*) Left transverse view of the thyroid superior pole with cricoid and tracheal pressure demonstrating significant lateralization of the hypoechoic mass.

parathyroid exploration resulted in the discovery of a superior parathyroid adenoma that was quite large, weighing 2.0 g and measuring 1.8 × 1.4 × 1.0 cm. The preoperative imaging included an equivocal sestamibi scan and an indistinct mass seen posterior to the midportion of the thyroid gland on a diagnostic ultrasound performed in the radiology suite. In the operating room, after the patient was intubated and positioned, a rapid ultrasound evaluation of the neck was undertaken. During this evaluation, pressure was applied to the cricoid and trachea at different points. Intraoperatively, surgeons frequently apply tracheal pressure to attempt to lateralize medially positioned and true retroesophageal parathyroids during palpation of the neck contents. During the preincision ultrasound, when pressure was applied, a very evident hypoechoic mass located about the level of the cricoid presented posterolateral to the thyroid (see **Fig. 6**). The surgical exploration amply demonstrated the mobility of the gland, an attribute that could have had real-world consequences and potentially resulted in a failed exploration. As the thyroid was rotated, no mass was evident, even as the exploration was carried well into the tracheoesophageal groove with identification of the recurrent laryngeal nerve just below the cricothyroid joint. It was only after pressure was applied to the trachea that a mass pooched out posterior and medial to the nerve. The relatively large parathyroid adenoma was able to assume a full retropharyngeal position because of the retraction of the thyroid and trachea. The immediate preoperative ultrasound had predicted for it and aided the surgical exploration.

Preincision ultrasound lymph node localization can also be very helpful to the operating surgeon. Metastatic papillary carcinoma is a common disease, and neck recurrence is a common scenario.[30] It has often been said that well-differentiated thyroid carcinoma is a disease of morbidity and not mortality because of the frequency of recurrences over a relatively normal lifespan, which most patients can expect. Proper decision making with regard to neck dissection is important because of the morbidity of more extended procedures and the lack of clear improvement in treatment outcomes when performing prophylactic neck dissections in the N0 neck when treating well-differentiated thyroid carcinoma.[30–32] This lack of difference in outcomes extends to comparisons of node plucking for palpable neck masses and selective neck dissections.[33] The only significant difference seems to be in regional recurrence rates. Based on the available data, general opinions on when to do elective neck dissections for well-differentiated thyroid cancer run the full gamut from never to always, whereas the biggest argument for prophylactic neck dissection in the N0 neck seems to be to forestall recurrence. In order to maximize benefits versus risks, an argument can be made for superselective neck dissections (eg, levels III/IV only) to remove just the suspicious nodes harboring early macroscopic disease.

Ultrasound for the N0 Neck

The increasing use of ultrasound is effectively moving the bar on what traditionally has been called an N0 neck. Ultrasound has proven to be the most sensitive imaging modality for detecting suspicious lateral neck nodes.[34] The characteristic findings of shape change, loss of the normal internal structure, and change in blood flow all contribute to the identification of metastatic nodes as small as 3 mm.[35,36] The latest guidelines from the American Thyroid Association (ATA) reflect the growing emphasis on using ultrasound as the primary modality to follow previously treated patients.[15] The routine use of thyroglobulin levels and nuclear medicine imaging with or without serial ultrasounds has also made the discovery of suspicious subcentimeter nodes more frequent in this group.[37] Whether and when to treat persistent, small, macroscopic disease is an on-going debate in the thyroid cancer literature. The discovery of highly suspicious nodes is difficult for patients and their endocrinologist to just observe, leading to increasing requests for selective neck dissections and reoperations.

Intraoperative Localization of Lymph Nodes

Properly removing subcentimeter disease in an adequate fashion is a dilemma for the operating surgeon. Intraoperative localization of small lymph nodes can be difficult based on palpation and visual clues alone. Until recently, the use of neck compartment nomenclature has not been widely used in radiology reports.[15] In the experience of the author, the most common localization descriptions have been limited to the upper neck, lower neck, lateral neck, and central neck. This circumstance is starting to change based on the recommendations accepted by the sonography groups and the ATA's guidelines,[15] but the interpretation of the neck compartments is still subject to variability both in the understanding of what the landmarks are as well as the effects of flexible neck structures. With regard to the former issue, the defined landmarks include structures with which the nonsurgeon sonographer is typically unfamiliar, such as the hyoid bone dividing level II and level III. The default behavior is to divide all necks roughly into 3 sections with the attendant ambiguities between levels II and IV and the combining of level I and level II. The position of the neck can significantly alter the attribution of lymph nodes between levels II and IV and level V located posterior to the sternocleidomastoid muscle.

Head and Neck Anatomic Landmarks

With respect to understanding and using anatomic landmarks, the operative head and neck surgeon is without equal. Reviewing the cineloop included with any well-done diagnostic ultrasound can place suspicious nodes with respect to ultrasound-discernable structures, including the internal jugular vein, carotid artery, sternocleidomastoid muscle, and the omohyoid muscle (**Fig. 7**). The omohyoid muscle is an easily appreciated landmark on cineloops as well as on appropriate still images (see **Fig. 7**)

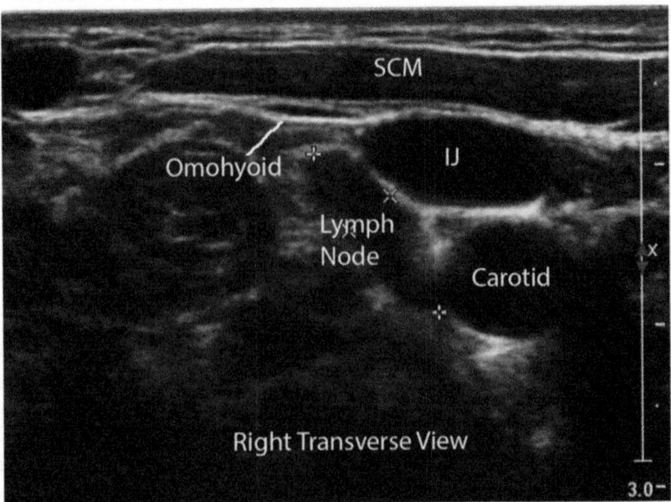

Fig. 7. Right neck transverse view of an abnormal lymph node measuring 1.3 × 0.9 × 0.4 cm. The node is posterior to the internal jugular vein (IJ) and carotid artery in level IV. The omohyoid muscle slip is visible posterior and superficial to the IJ, just deep to the sternocleidomastoid muscle (SCM).

and is an important landmark for the operating surgeon. Likewise, the surgeon can easily appreciate the position of nodes with respect to the vascular structures. Although this information can be gleaned from the preoperative images, postpositioning ultrasound allows the operating surgeon to locate the suspicious nodes with respect to palpable structures, including the hyoid, the thyroid and cricoid cartilages, and the clavicles. This type of information can prove invaluable in designing neck incisions and defining the boundaries of the selective neck dissection.

FURTHER READINGS

There are many books available that are invaluable resources to the neophyte ultrasonographer as well as the experienced nonradiologist ultrasonographer. The author has listed 3 books here that are highly readable and aimed specifically at the head and neck surgical practitioner. They range in price and comprehensiveness. Two of the volumes include DVDs or refer to online resources, including cineloops.

Anil A, Evans R, editors. Practical head and neck ultrasound. London: Greenwich Medical Media Ltd; 2000.

Orloff LA, editor. Head and neck ultrasonography. San Diego (CA): Plural Publishing; 2008.

Sofferman RA, Ahuja AT, editors. Ultrasound of the thyroid and parathyroid glands. New York: Springer; 2012.

REFERENCES

1. AAO-HNS bulletin, page 28, September 2013.
2. Short MW, Jorgensen JE, Edwards JA, et al. Assessing intern core competencies with an objective structured clinical examination. J Grad Med Educ 2009;1:30–6.
3. Kasales CJ, Coulson CC, Mauger D, et al. Training in obstetric sonography for radiology residents and fellows in the United States. Am J Roentgenol 2001; 177:763–7.
4. Mandavia DP, Aragona J, Chan L, et al. Henderson SO ultrasound training for emergency physicians - a prospective study. Acad Emerg Med 2000;7:1008–14.
5. Rozycki GS. Surgeon-performed ultrasound: its use in clinical practice. Ann Surg 1998;228:16–28.
6. McCarter FD, Luchette FA, Molloy M, et al. Institutional and individual learning curves for focused abdominal ultrasound for trauma cumulative sum analysis. Ann Surg 2000;231:689–700.
7. Moon HJ, Kim EK, Yoon JH, et al. Differences in the diagnostic performances of staging US for thyroid malignancy according to experience. Ultrasound Med Biol 2012;38(4):568–73.
8. Hertzberg BS, Kliewer MA, Bowie JD, et al. Physician training requirements in sonography: how many cases are needed for competence? Am J Roentgenol 2000; 174:1221–7.
9. Medical ultrasound equipment - global strategic business report. Research and markets, Report 338878, October 2011.
10. Nagarkatti S, Merkel M, Sofferman R, et al. Overcoming obstacles to setting up office-based ultrasound for evaluation of thyroid and parathyroid disorders. Laryngoscope 2011;121:1–7.
11. Matt BH, Butler PD, Woodward-Hagg HK, et al. Lean six sigma applied to ultrasound of the head and neck: changing patient management. Otolaryngol Head Neck Surg 2013;149(No. 2 Suppl):68–9.

12. Mazzaferri EL. Management of a solitary thyroid nodule. N Engl J Med 1993;328: 553–9.
13. Mazzaferri EL, de los Santos ET, Rofagha-Keyhani S. Solitary thyroid nodule: diagnosis and management. Med Clin North Am 1988;72:1177–211.
14. Pelizzo MR, Piotto A, Rubello D, et al. High prevalence of occult papillary carcinoma in a surgical series of benign thyroid disease. Tumori 1990;76:255–7.
15. Cooper DS, Doherty GM, Haugen BR, et al. Revised American Thyroid Association management guidelines for patients with thyroid nodules and differentiated thyroid cancer. Thyroid 2009;11:1–48.
16. Gharib H, Papini E, Valcavi R, et al. American Association of Clinical Endocrinologists and Associazione Medici Endocrinologi medical guidelines for clinical practice for the diagnosis and management of thyroid nodules. Endocr Pract 2006;12:63–102.
17. Kim EK, Park CS, Chung WY, et al. New sonographic criteria for recommending fine-needle aspiration biopsy of nonpalpable solid nodules of the thyroid. Am J Roentgenol 2002;178:687–91.
18. Frates MC, Benson CB, Charboneau JW, et al. Management of thyroid nodules detected at US: Society of Radiologists in Ultrasound consensus conference statement. Radiology 2005;237:794–800.
19. Frates MC, Langer J. Letter to editor regarding- Biopsy of thyroid nodules: comparison of three sets of guidelines. Am J Roentgenol 2010;195:W472.
20. Ahn SS, Kim E, Kang DR, et al. Biopsy of thyroid nodules: comparison of three sets of guidelines. Am J Roentgenol 2010;194:31–7.
21. Kim HG, Moon HJ, Kwak JY, et al. Diagnostic accuracy of the ultrasonographic features for subcentimeter thyroid nodules suggested by the revised American Thyroid Association guidelines. Thyroid 2013;23(12):1583–9.
22. Chan BK, Desser TS, McDougall R, et al. Common and uncommon sonographic features of papillary thyroid carcinoma. J Ultrasound Med 2003;22:1083–90.
23. Cappelli C, Castellano M, Pirola I, et al. The predictive value of ultrasound findings in the management of thyroid nodules. QJM 2007;100:29–35.
24. Frates MC, Benson CB, Doubilet PM, et al. Prevalence and distribution of carcinoma in patients with solitary and multiple thyroid nodules on sonography. J Clin Endocrinol Metab 2006;91:3411–7.
25. Moon WJ, Jung SL, Lee JH, et al. Benign and malignant thyroid nodules: US differentiation— multicenter retrospective study. Radiology 2008;247:762–70.
26. Nam-Goong IS, Kim HY, Gong G, et al. Ultrasonography-guided fine-needle aspiration of thyroid incidentaloma: correlation with pathological findings. Clin Endocrinol (Oxf) 2004;60:21–8.
27. Papini E, Guglielmi R, Bianchini A, et al. Risk of malignancy in nonpalpable thyroid nodules: predictive value of ultrasound and color-Doppler features. J Clin Endocrinol Metab 2002;87:1941–6.
28. Cap J, Ryska A, Rehorkova P, et al. Sensitivity and specificity of the fine needle aspiration biopsy of the thyroid: clinical point of view. Clin Endocrinol (Oxf) 1999; 51:509–15.
29. Miccoli P, Berti P, Raffaelli M, et al. Comparison between minimally invasive video-assisted thyroidectomy and conventional thyroidectomy: a prospective randomized study. Surgery 2001;130:1039–43.
30. Mazzaferri EL, Jhiang AM. Long-term impact of initial surgical and medical therapy on papillary and follicular thyroid cancer. Am J Med 1994;97:418–28.
31. Sivanandan R, Soo KC. Pattern of cervical lymph node metastases from papillary carcinoma of the thyroid. Br J Surg 2001;88:1241–4.

32. Qubain SW, Nakano S, Baba M, et al. Distribution of lymph node micrometastasis in pN0 well-differentiated thyroid carcinoma. Surgery 2002;131:249–56.
33. Mazzaferri EL, Kloos RT. Current approaches to primary therapy for papillary carcinoma and follicular cancer. J Clin Endocrinol Metab 2001;86:1447–64.
34. Choi JS, Kim J, Kwak JY, et al. Preoperative staging of papillary thyroid carcinoma: comparison of ultrasound imaging and CT. Am J Roentgenol 2009;193:871–8.
35. Ahuja A, Ying M. Sonography of neck lymph nodes. Part II: abnormal lymph nodes. Clin Radiol 2003;58:359–66.
36. Mittendorf EA, Wang X, Perrier ND, et al. Follow up of patients with papillary thyroid cancer: in search of the optimal algorithm. J Am Coll Surg 2007;205:239–47.
37. Franceschi M, Kusic Z, Franceschi D, et al. Thyroglobulin determination, neck ultrasonography and iodine-131 whole-body scintigraphy in differentiated thyroid carcinoma. J Nucl Med 1996;37:446–51.

Clinician-Performed Thyroid Ultrasound-Guided Fine-Needle Aspiration

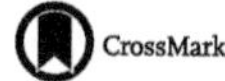

Gabriel J. Tsao, MD[a], Lisa A. Orloff, MD[b,*]

KEYWORDS

• Thyroid • Ultrasound • Biopsy • Fine-needle aspiration • FNA

KEY POINTS

- Although palpation-guided fine-needle aspiration (FNA) continues to be a successful approach to the evaluation of palpable lesions, ultrasound-guided FNA (USGFNA) enhances precision, documentation, and diagnostic yield in nonpalpable, and even in palpable, masses.
- Both long-axis (parallel) and short-axis (perpendicular) approaches to performing USGFNA should be available, because certain lesions and conditions lend themselves better to one approach than the other.
- A consistent, step-by-step approach to performing USGFNA and collaboration with one's cytopathology colleagues will lead to the greatest diagnostic success in the management of thyroid pathology.

Videos of ultrasound-guided fine-needle aspiration accompany this article at http://www.oto.theclinics.com/

INTRODUCTION

Fine-needle aspiration (FNA) biopsy is an indispensable component of the evaluation and management of thyroid pathology. Since its widespread adoption in the 1980s, it has come to be recognized as the gold standard for evaluation of a thyroid nodule. Traditionally, FNA has been used to obtain cells for cytologic diagnosis, supplemented by immunocytochemistry. More recently, as noted in later articles in this issue, FNA has been used to obtain material for genetic and molecular testing. FNA also is useful for obtaining tissue samples for chemical testing, and the same techniques used for

---

Financial disclosures of conflicts of interest: None.

[a] Department of Otolaryngology–Head and Neck Surgery, University of California, San Francisco, 2380 Sutter Street, 2nd Floor, San Francisco, CA 94115, USA; [b] Division of Head and Neck and Endocrine Surgery, Department of Otolaryngology–Head and Neck Surgery, University of California, San Francisco, 875 Blake Wilbur Drive, CC-2225, Stanford, CA 94305-5826, USA
* Corresponding author. Division of Head and Neck and Endocrine Surgery, Department of Otolaryngology–Head and Neck Surgery, Stanford University, 875 Blake Wilbur Drive CC-2225, Stanford, CA 94305-5826, USA.
E-mail address: lorloff@ohns.stanford.edu

Otolaryngol Clin N Am 47 (2014) 509–518
http://dx.doi.org/10.1016/j.otc.2014.04.005 oto.theclinics.com
0030-6665/14/$ – see front matter

Abbreviations	
FNA	Fine-needle aspiration
US	Ultrasound
USGFNA	Ultrasound-guided fine-needle aspiration

diagnostic FNA can be applied to needle placement for a variety of therapeutic procedures. The application of ultrasound (US) technology to FNA is useful for biopsy of nonpalpable and even palpable nodules, and enhances precision, feedback, and documentation to the FNA and other needle-placement procedures.

ULTRASOUND-GUIDED FNA

FNA biopsy is a critical step in the evaluation of thyroid and related neck masses. Although the acronym FNA has persisted and implies a component of aspiration, the procedure is more accurately described as FNB, or fine-needle biopsy, as aspiration is not a requirement. Traditionally, FNA is performed by method of manual palpation. The size threshold for palpating thyroid nodules is 1.5 to 2.0 cm, and up to 30% of FNA biopsies without ultrasound guidance can be nondiagnostic.[1] The introduction of US guidance to thyroid FNA has reduced the number of inadequate samples by half, from 8.7% to 16.0% down to 3.5% to 7.0%.[2–5] US in conjunction with US-guided FNA (USGFNA) also has been shown to assist in identification of suspicious nodules that should be sampled.[1,6] Not uncommonly, the most suspicious nodule on US for malignancy is not the largest nodule, and if only dominant (by size) or palpable nodules were aspirated, malignancy could easily be missed. In one series, patients given benign diagnoses based on palpation-guided FNA were reevaluated with USGFNA, resulting in 14% reclassification to diagnoses of malignancies.[7] The accuracy, sensitivity, and specificity of USGFNA, reported at 80%, 83%, and 77%, respectively, is improved compared with palpation-guided FNA.[8]

After FNA is performed, specimens are reviewed by a cytopathologist. On-site evaluation by a team composed of clinical physicians and pathologists has been shown to provide the most accurate results, while at the same time reducing patient discomfort.[5,9,10] Reduction of patient discomfort is achieved by leveraging US guidance to limit the number of needle passes required and improve sampling adequacy rate, as well as provide immediate examination of the material obtained so as not to require multiple separate sampling procedures. In this instance, a desktop or portable microscope must be available for slide review (**Fig. 1**). In part because of these advantages, immediate on-site pathologic evaluation has been strongly advocated by some as the standard of care.[5,9,10] However, a study by Bhatki and colleagues[11] demonstrated that on-site cytologic specimen evaluation was not necessary to confirm cytologic adequacy; that a combination of experienced USGFNA and 3 to 4 needle passes produce comparable results while conserving costs and resources. Also, for practical and cost-effective purposes, FNA without US guidance still may be appropriate or preferable for palpable thyroid masses.

THYROID FNA BIOPSY

A detailed description of cytologic findings in benign and malignant thyroid disease can be found in an earlier article. However, certain preliminary findings can suggest specimen adequacy as well as a diagnosis. Benign thyroid nodules often yield grossly visible watery or viscous colloid material in addition to microscopic clusters of follicular cells in a monolayer or "honeycombed" pattern, and round to oval nuclei with

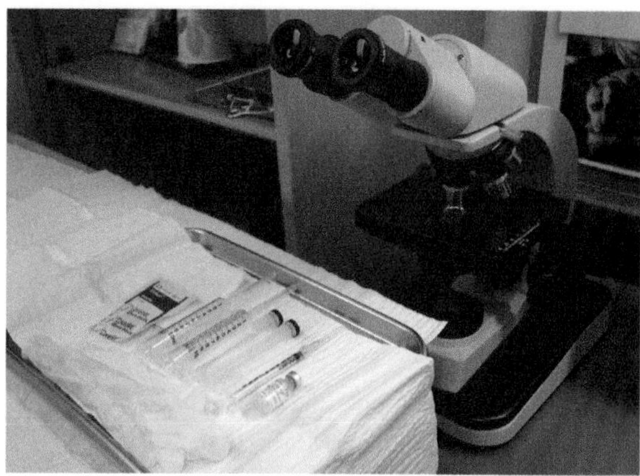

Fig. 1. Procedure room set-up with tray of simple supplies for USGFNA and desktop microscope. Supplies include 25-gauge needles with syringes, 1% lidocaine with injection needle and syringe, 4 × 4 gauze, alcohol swabs, adhesive bandage, and nonsterile gloves. Not shown are glass slides and fixative(s).

uniform chromatin and foamy (degenerating) cells.[12] In addition to the cytologic features of subacute thyroiditis (de Quervain thyroiditis) that include scant colloid, giant cells, mixed inflammatory background (depending on early vs late stage),[13] a very painful FNA procedure may be an additional clue to this diagnosis.

Follicular patterned lesions are a cytopathological dilemma, as they cannot distinguish between benign and malignant nonpapillary follicular and Hurthle cell lesions. Surgical excision and histopathological analysis for vascular or capsular invasion have traditionally been necessary in these cases to give a definitive diagnosis.[14,15] In our experience, FNA of follicular neoplasms tends to be bloodier than FNA of other thyroid lesions.

TECHNICAL ASPECTS OF USGFNA

FNA techniques vary between individuals and institutions, yet there are several common components that are universal. In this section, we aim to evaluate modifications, including US guidance, that can improve the diagnostic success of FNA. A step-by-step guide is presented in **Box 1**. US guidance allows the practitioner to visualize the tip of the needle as it passes through tissue, ensuring that the cells examined are indeed from the intended area. Orienting the bevel of the needle toward the US transducer improves visualization of the needle tip. Even within a target lesion, there are areas that may give a higher diagnostic yield when biopsied, such as the solid component of a mixed solid-cystic nodule. An area of initial hemorrhage from a first pass on USGFNA also can be avoided on subsequent passes.

Informed consent should be obtained before the procedure. The most significant possible complication is the development of a neck hematoma, but this complication is exceptionally rare. The patient should be questioned for a history of anticoagulant therapy, such as warfarin or aspirin, although it is rarely necessary to discontinue such medication before the biopsy. In general, only if there has been a previous unsuccessful USGFNA while the patient was taking anticoagulation therapy should USGFNA be repeated with an adequate interval of discontinuation of anticoagulation therapy.

When possible, the patient is placed in the supine position with the neck slightly extended. The head can be turned to improve visualization and access to the target

Box 1
Ultrasound-guided fine-needle aspiration (USGFNA): step-by-step procedure

- Diagnostic ultrasound complete
- Target lesion reconfirmed, may mark needle entry site with surgical marking pen
- Informed consent obtained, perform Time Out.
- Local anesthesia administered
- "Prep and drape"
- Room lighting off (except small backlight)
- USGFNA:
  - Transducer in nondominant hand, needle in dominant hand
  - Insert needle into lesion under ultrasound visualization
  - Traverse diameter of lesion multiple, times until flash in hub of needle
  - Withdraw needle and apply direct pressure with gauze (transfer pressure-holding to patient)
  - Hit "Freeze" on ultrasound system
  - Eject specimen onto slide and smear (or pass to cytopathologist/tech)
  - Rinse needle for immunohistochemistry/chemistry/flow cytometry
  - Annotate and save video for documentation
  - Repeat with new needles as necessary for additional passes
- Apply bandage to skin

lesion. Both patient and operator should be comfortable during the procedure. Depending on the location of the lesion, the operator may stand or sit at the patient's side or at the head. Although diagnostic US uses conventional transverse and sagittal planes for imaging, once a lesion has been visualized and targeted for FNA, the transducer can be oriented in any position that will better facilitate the procedure. For instance, to approach a lesion in the left lobe of the thyroid, a right-handed operator may prefer to stand at the patient's head to approach the lesion from the trachea side as opposed to the carotid side, thus performing the procedure "upside-down." Many US devices have special features to assist practitioners in USGFNA. Some have attachable needle guides, but these tend to be discouraged by experienced clinicians, as they are an added expense and they limit flexibility in biopsy direction.

The issue of sterility during US-guided office-based procedures can be regarded as similar to the sterility recommended for phlebotomy. Preparations range from a simple hand-washing and no transducer cover to an iodine-based skin disinfectant, use of sterile aqueous jelly, and a sterile transducer cover. A reasonable compromise involves the use of an alcohol-based skin disinfectant and nonsterile aqueous gel applied to the footprint of the transducer before and after its coverage with a plastic wrap or disposable glove secured with a rubber band (**Fig. 2**). These inexpensive techniques have been used extensively by the senior author (LAO) and infectious complications have not been encountered.

The use of local anesthesia is not universal, but most experienced physicians use local anesthesia for thyroid FNAs,[16] given its low-risk profile and reduction of discomfort, which reduces patient movement. We use a small amount (<1.0 mL) of 1% lidocaine without epinephrine within the dermis and subcutaneous tissues. Care should be taken

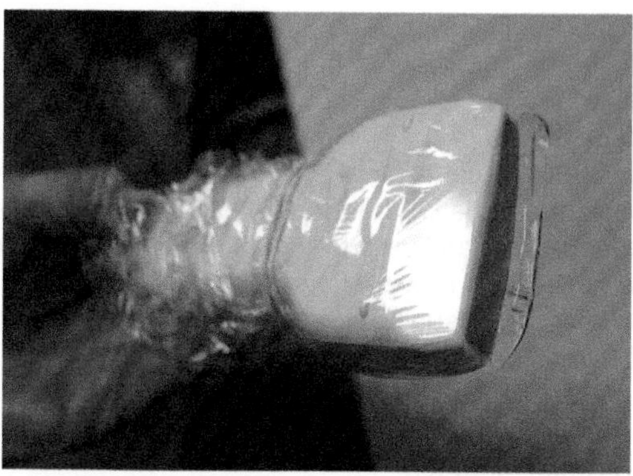

Fig. 2. US transducer prepared for USGFNA by applying thin layer of gel followed by plastic wrap and then an additional thin layer of gel (or as an alternative, alcohol).

not to inject excessive amounts of anesthesia close to the target lesion, as dilution of the aspirate can occur and aggressive injection can increase the risk of a bloody aspirate.

Historically, "core needles," such as those in the range of 14 to 19 gauge, were used in needle biopsy. A comparison of FNA with core-needle biopsy was performed in a prospective study demonstrating that the diagnostic yield with core-needle biopsy of thyroid nodules exceeded that with FNA techniques by approximately 10%.[17] Another study demonstrated a higher adequacy rate with core-needle biopsy but decreased sensitivity, especially for papillary thyroid carcinoma.[18] Predictably, there also was a higher complication rate with the use of core needles. FNA remains the best technique available to date for the initial evaluation of thyroid nodules. The slight increase in diagnostic accuracy from core-needle biopsy is outweighed by the reduced hematoma rates, decreased bloody aspirates, improved patient comfort, and theoretical reduction in the rate of malignant dissemination.[19,20] We favor the use of 1.5-inch (38-mm) length, 25-gauge needles, or longer (40–50 mm) needles for lesions at greater depth. Calcified masses may be more amenable to biopsy with a finer needle, such as a 27 gauge. Larger-diameter needles are generally reserved for drainage of viscous colloid cyst contents or considered for patients in whom initial FNA yields only scant-appearing cellularity or after prior failed FNA.

There are 2 approaches that can be used with respect to orienting the biopsy needle with the US transducer: the long-axis or parallel approach, and the short-axis or perpendicular approach (**Fig. 3**; see **Fig. 5**). With the long-axis approach, the needle

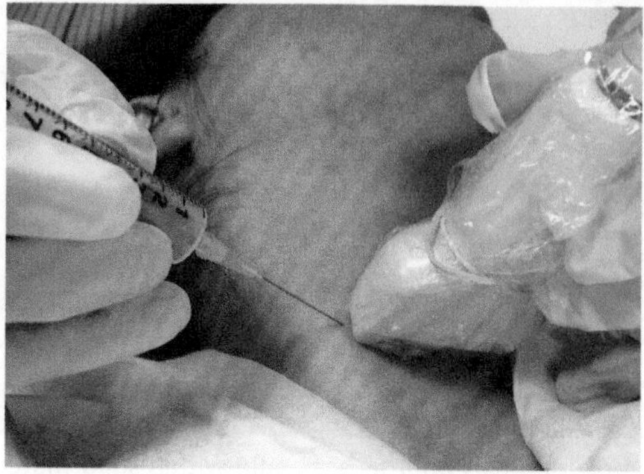

Fig. 3. USGFNA orientation for long-axis approach.

is inserted just adjacent to the midpoint of the far end of the transducer, and exactly parallel to it at a 45-degree angle ideally (this angle can range from 30 to 70 degrees, depending on the depth of the target and the length of the needle) (see **Fig. 3**). This approach allows visualization of the entire length of the needle and its trajectory as it advances toward and into the lesion (**Fig. 4**, Video 1). The needle advances deep to and in-plane or parallel to the US beam. Alternatively, the short-axis approach involves placing the needle just adjacent to the midpoint of the full width of the transducer, aligned with its handle, in a perpendicular fashion (**Fig. 5**). A nearly vertical trajectory is used to maintain visualization of the lesion and one will see only the tip of the needle as a bright spot as it crosses under the US beam in a perpendicular trajectory and arrives at the plane of the target (Video 2). It is advisable to be comfortable with both techniques, as there are times when lesion location and accessibility will favor one approach versus another.

One can use the capillary or the aspiration method of needle biopsy for collecting the sample. Studies comparing FNA with and without aspiration have shown no difference between the 2 techniques with regard to diagnostic accuracy.[21] The increased surface tension within smaller needle diameters offers an innate suction mechanism such that aspiration on the needle is frequently not necessary. During the biopsy, the needle is held free or attached to an empty syringe with the plunger removed. After the pass is completed, the plunger is reinserted or a syringe is attached to the needle to expel the sample onto the slide. If the aspiration method is preferred, a number of syringe holders are commercially available to assist in the procedure. Advocates of the syringe method report increased amounts of sample per pass, but aspiration also may increase the amount of extraneous tissue and blood within the specimen. If aspiration is used, it is important to apply suction only once within the target tissue and discontinue suction before exiting the target to reduce specimen contamination. Some operators prefer a combination of the 2 techniques, with the capillary method for the first pass followed by the aspiration technique for subsequent passes.[11] It is advisable, as with most topics in this article, to discuss the FNA preferences of your cytopathologist when deciding on a biopsy technique.

Using either the short-axis or long-axis technique, the needle is advanced into the target lesion under US guidance (**Fig. 6**). Once visualized within the target lesion,

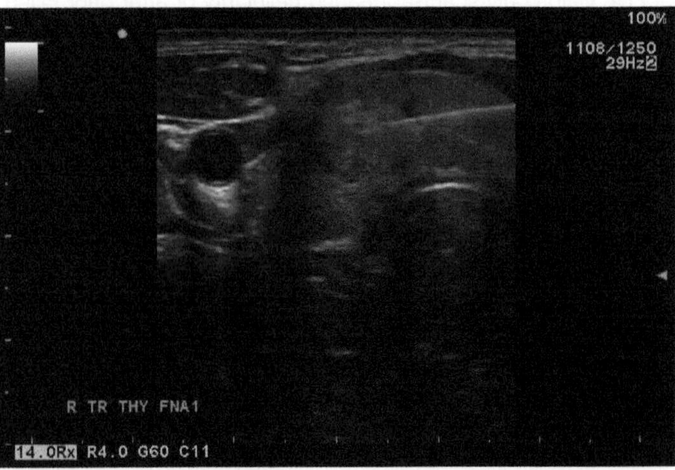

Fig. 4. Still US image of long-axis approach: needle within solid material within complex cystic thyroid nodule.

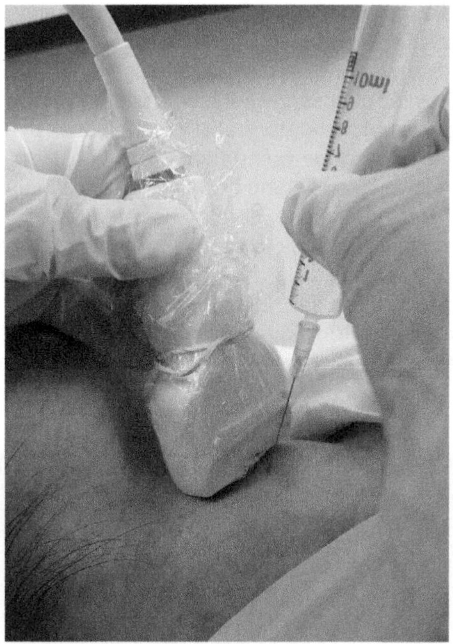

Fig. 5. USGFNA orientation for short-axis approach.

the needle is oscillated forward and backward at a rate of 2 cycles per second for a dwell time between 3 and 10 seconds. This interval maximizes cellular yield, minimizes bloody artifacts, and efficiently produces 1 to 2 slides per biopsy pass. With this back-and-forth movement, the free needle edge shaves cells from within the mass. Once a pink flash is visualized in the needle hub, the needle is removed. Occasionally, no flash is observed, but after approximately 20 excursions (~10 seconds) it is appropriate to withdraw the needle.

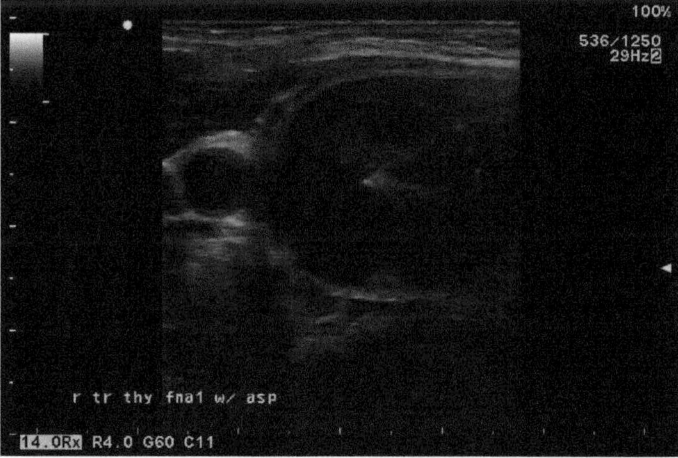

Fig. 6. Still US image of long-axis approach: needle within solid thyroid nodule that proved to be a follicular lesion by cytology.

The number of needle passes needed for cytologic adequacy has been extensively researched and debated.[5,22] If a needle is clearly visualized within the area of interest, one pass may be sufficient. An on-site cytopathologist can review the adequacy of the specimen immediately, and if necessary, additional passes can be made. As mentioned earlier, on-site pathology is not mandatory, and a combination of experienced USGFNA and 3 to 4 needle passes produce comparable results.[11] Additional needle passes may potentially cause increased bleeding and decrease the diagnostic yield of subsequent passes. Nevertheless, US guidance may assist in the redirection of the biopsy needle away from prior pass locations toward more preferred sites within the lesion.

Different preparations, such as the Papanicolaou staining method or the Diff-Quik/Giemsa stains, are commonly used. When the Papanicolaou staining method is used, the smears should be quickly placed in 95% alcohol for fixation. When Diff-Quik or Giemsa stain is used, the smear should simply be allowed to air dry. Direct

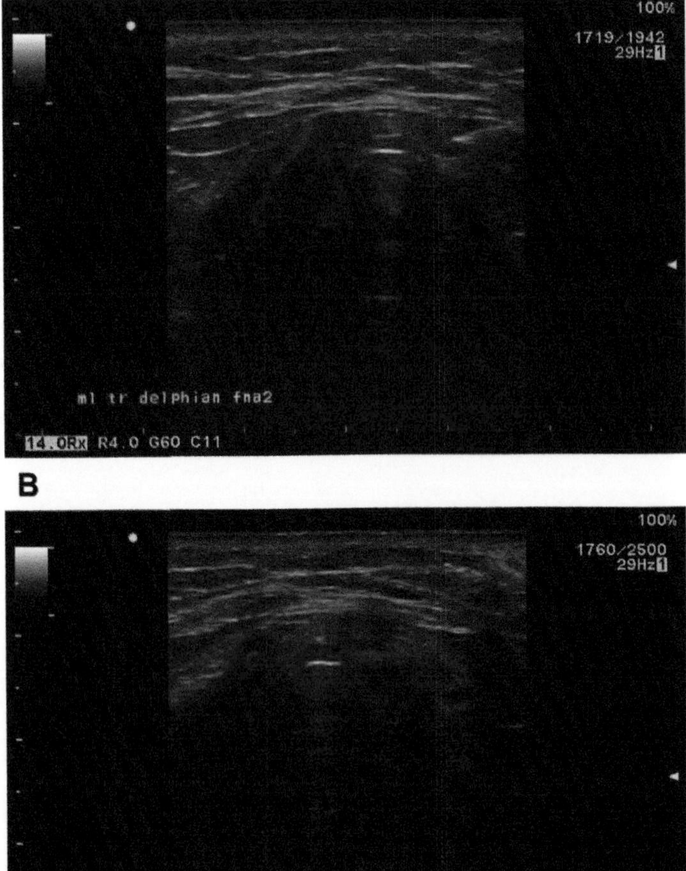

Fig. 7. Still US images of both long-axis (*A*) and short-axis (*B*) approaches to the same target; note needle within Delphian lymph node (same patient and target as Videos 3 and 4).

smears can be processed alone or with a liquid-based cytology and/or a supplemental cell block. Papanicolaou staining is most commonly used for cytologic analysis of thyroid specimens, and it provides the clearest depiction of nuclear chromatin, ground-glass nuclei, and nuclear grooves characteristic of papillary carcinoma. Diff-Quik or Giemsa stain help visualize the characteristics of cytoplasm and colloid.[23] In cases of suspected lymphoma, samples also should be obtained for flow cytometry, which requires an abundance of cells that are typically rinsed in RPMI medium. If immunocytochemistry is anticipated, needles also should be rinsed in formalin to obtain a sample for cell block. Of note, US gel can get admixed with the cytologic sample and create confusion for the cytopathologist, even though experienced cytopathologists can recognize this inorganic material readily. Therefore, during sample collection and preparation, it is wise to minimize the presence of gel in the pathway of the needle.

USGFNA of extrathyroidal targets is performed in a manner identical to that of thyroid lesions, yet the regional anatomy differs and may therefore necessitate alternative orientations of the transducer and the needle trajectory (**Fig. 7**, Videos 3 and 4). The FNA procedure is otherwise performed in the same step-by-step fashion described in **Box 1**. In addition to cytologic assessment, the aspirated material can be tested for thyroglobulin and calcitonin levels. These assays are particularly useful in confirming tissue of thyroid origin within lymph nodes or the thyroid bed indicative of metastasis or recurrent disease. These levels should be correlated with simultaneous serum levels. Serum thyroglobulin and calcitonin levels are commonly monitored as a marker for recurrence. Measurements of thyroglobulin or calcitonin in FNA specimens can confirm the presence of disease and simultaneously assist in its localization. Similarly, aspirated material can be processed for molecular or genetic studies (as described in the articles by Ferris and colleagues, Kloos and colleagues, and Tufano and colleagues elsewhere in this issue) whether the source is from within or outside of the thyroid itself.

SUMMARY

The use of US to guide FNA of the thyroid and related structures of the neck, in addition to guiding other interventional procedures as needed, provides precision with increased anatomic visualization and decreased guesswork. USGFNA is a logical extension of diagnostic US, and the techniques and pearls described herein are intended to assist the clinician in optimizing the diagnostic evaluation of patients with thyroid pathology.

SUPPLEMENTARY DATA

Supplementary data related to this article can be found online at http://dx.doi.org/10.1016/j.otc.2014.04.005.

REFERENCES

1. Papini E, Guglielmi R, Bianchini A, et al. Risk of malignancy in nonpalpable thyroid nodules: predictive value of ultrasound and color-Doppler features. J Clin Endocrinol Metab 2002;87:1941–6.
2. Carmeci C, Jeffrey RB, McDougall IR, et al. Ultrasound-guided fine-needle aspiration biopsy of thyroid masses. Thyroid 1998;8:283–9.
3. Cesur M, Corapcioglu D, Bulut S, et al. Comparison of palpation-guided fine-needle aspiration biopsy to ultrasound-guided fine-needle aspiration biopsy in the evaluation of thyroid nodules. Thyroid 2006;16:555–61.

4. Danese D, Sciacchitano S, Farsetti A, et al. Diagnostic accuracy of conventional versus sonography-guided fine-needle aspiration biopsy of thyroid nodules. Thyroid 1998;8:15–21.
5. Redman R, Zalaznick H, Mazzaferri EL, et al. The impact of assessing specimen adequacy and number of needle passes for fine-needle aspiration biopsy of thyroid nodules. Thyroid 2006;16:55–60.
6. Deandrea M, Mormile A, Veglio M, et al. Fine-needle aspiration biopsy of the thyroid: comparison between thyroid palpation and ultrasonography. Endocr Pract 2002;8:282–6.
7. Yokozawa T, Fukata S, Kuma K, et al. Thyroid cancer detected by ultrasound-guided fine-needle aspiration biopsy. World J Surg 1996;20:848–53 [discussion: 853].
8. Karstrup S, Balslev E, Juul N, et al. US-guided fine needle aspiration versus coarse needle biopsy of thyroid nodules. Eur J Ultrasound 2001;13:1–5.
9. Baloch ZW, Tam D, Langer J, et al. Ultrasound-guided fine-needle aspiration biopsy of the thyroid: role of on-site assessment and multiple cytologic preparations. Diagn Cytopathol 2000;23:425–9.
10. Zhu W, Michael CW. How important is on-site adequacy assessment for thyroid FNA? An evaluation of 883 cases. Diagn Cytopathol 2007;35:183–6.
11. Bhatki AM, Brewer B, Robinson-Smith T, et al. Adequacy of surgeon-performed ultrasound-guided thyroid fine-needle aspiration biopsy. Otolaryngol Head Neck Surg 2008;139:27–31.
12. Kini SR, editor. Guides to clinical aspiration biopsy thyroid. New York: Igaku-Shoin; 1996.
13. Gharib H. Thyroid fine needle aspiration biopsy. Boston: Kluwer Academic Publ; 2000.
14. Kumar N, Ray C, Jain S. Aspiration cytology of Hashimoto's thyroiditis in an endemic area. Cytopathology 2002;13:31–9.
15. Kumarasinghe MP, De Silva S. Pitfalls in cytological diagnosis of autoimmune thyroiditis. Pathology 1999;31:1–7.
16. Gharib H, Goellner JR. Fine-needle aspiration biopsy of the thyroid: an appraisal [see comments]. Ann Intern Med 1993;4:282–9.
17. Quinn SF, Nelson HA, Demlow TA. Thyroid biopsies: fine-needle aspiration biopsy versus spring-activated core biopsy needle in 102 patients. J Vasc Interv Radiol 1994;5:619–23.
18. Renshaw AA, Pinnar N. Comparison of thyroid fine-needle aspiration and core needle biopsy. Am J Clin Pathol 2007;128:370–4.
19. Degirmenci B, Haktanir A, Albayrak R, et al. Sonographically guided fine-needle biopsy of thyroid nodules: the effects of nodule characteristics, sampling technique, and needle size on the adequacy of cytological material. Clin Radiol 2007;62:798–803.
20. Lo Gerfo P, Colacchio T, Caushaj F, et al. Comparison of fine-needle and coarse-needle biopsies in evaluating thyroid nodules. Surgery 1982;92:835–8.
21. Kate MS, Kamal MM, Bobhate SK, et al. Evaluation of fine needle capillary sampling in superficial and deep-seated lesions. An analysis of 670 cases. Acta Cytol 1998;42:679–84.
22. Hamburger JI, Husain M, Nishiyama R, et al. Increasing the accuracy of fine-needle biopsy for thyroid nodules. Arch Pathol Lab Med 1989;113:1035–41.
23. Oertel YC. Fine-needle aspiration of the thyroid: technique and terminology. Endocrinol Metab Clin North Am 2007;36:737–51, vi–vii.

Surgical Diagnosis

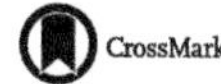

Frozen Section and the Extent of Surgery

Iain J. Nixon, PhD, Ashok R. Shaha, MD, Snehal G. Patel, MD*

KEYWORDS

• Thyroid cancer • Thyroidectomy • Neck dissection • Frozen section

KEY POINTS

- A surgical plan should be discussed preoperatively and based upon details of the clinical history, physical examination, and investigations.
- Patients with low-risk, intrathyroid disease should be offered thyroid lobectomy, while the remaining patients should be managed with total thyroidectomy.
- Patients with evidence of regional lymph node metastases should undergo systematic neck dissection, and patients considered without evidence of lymph node metastases (cN0) should not undergo elective lateral neck dissection.
- In the operating room, experience, clinical acumen, and frozen section should be used to adapt the surgical plan as required.
- With appropriate planning, low-risk patients will have survival rates greater than 95% at 10 years, and less than 50% of high-risk patients will die of disease.

OVERVIEW

Following preoperative investigation of thyroid cancer, which will involve ultrasound and cytologic assessment in most cases (as outlined elsewhere), the surgeon must decide upon an operative plan. This plan will be shaped by patient factors (such as age), ultrasonographic characteristics of the thyroid gland, thyroid nodules and associated regional lymph nodes, and the cytologic features of samples obtained (including presence of nuclear grooves and pseudoinclusions). Integration of these variables will allow the surgeon to assess the patient's risk of recurrence and death from disease. An appreciation of this risk, in conjunction with an understanding of disease biology, will allow the surgeon to recommend the plan most likely to maximize chances of surgical cure and minimize the potential for morbidity with a single procedure.

Disclosures: The authors have nothing to disclose.
Head and Neck Service, Department of Surgery, Memorial Sloan Kettering Cancer Center, 1275 York Avenue, New York, NY 10065, USA
* Corresponding author.
E-mail address: patels@mskcc.org

Otolaryngol Clin N Am 47 (2014) 519–528
http://dx.doi.org/10.1016/j.otc.2014.04.006
oto.theclinics.com

The aim of this article is to provide an understanding of the biology of well differentiated thyroid cancer (WDTC), and how relevant features of the patient and tumor impact on clinical risk and outcome. The authors go on to outline the procedures available for managing WDTC and the rationale for selecting appropriate therapy on an individual risk-stratified basis for both in relation to the thyroid gland and regional lymph nodes. The article concludes with an overview of the long-term outcomes that patients with WDTC can expect.

RELEVANT ANATOMY AND PATHOPHYSIOLOGY AND THEIR IMPACT ON RISK PREDICTION

WDTC is increasingly common, and papillary thyroid cancer is the most commonly encountered histologic subtype.[1–3] Indeed, over 80% of thyroid cancers are now considered papillary. Interestingly, autopsy studies show high rates of clinically undetected disease in patients who die of other causes, a finding that suggests that many lesions never impact on patient outcome during life.[4–6] Nonetheless, it is important to understand the pathology of this disease in order to make appropriate treatment decisions.

The increasing incidence of thyroid cancer is being driven in a large part by more intensive investigation of the US population. As such, the nature of the disease is changing. More patients with small-volume disease are presenting, and the average age at presentation is increasing. Today, the most commonly encountered thyroid cancer in the United States is a papillary carcinoma that measures less than 1 cm and has no detectable regional lymph node metastases.[7]

Outcomes for patients with WDTC are excellent.[1,8] Long-term follow-up of patients treated in many institutions confirms survival rates of over 90% at 10 years. The risk of recurrence and/or death can be estimated using a number of available systems based on patient and tumor factors.[9–13] Prior to considering these, some points about the nature of the disease should be considered.

Papillary thyroid cancer (PTC) has a propensity both for multifocality[14] and regional nodal metastasis.[15] Approximately 40% of PTC cases are multifocal (more than 1 PTC present in the thyroid gland). Although this has little impact on oncological outcome, preoperative investigation may identify bilateral nodules, which may be addressed with a single surgery. Extrathyroid extension (ETE) is extremely uncommon in disease less than 1 cm, and more common in larger-volume primary tumors.[16] Such ETE may be identified following clinical examination, on preoperative imaging, or on the operating table (gross ETE). This clinically apparent ETE has a significant impact, not only on rates of recurrence, but also on survival. In patients considered free of ETE following surgery, who have microscopic ETE on histopathological analysis, the impact is far less significant. Such patients are at higher risk of recurrence, but survival is unaffected by this finding.[17]

In terms of regional disease, PTC metastasizes often and early.[18] Even in those without clinical evidence of regional disease, occult metastases will be demonstrated in around 40% of patients if elective central and lateral neck surgery is performed.[15] These occult nodes do not confer worse survival, particularly in younger patients, and in most patients will never manifest clinically during follow-up. The prognosis in patients with evident regional metastases at presentation is influenced by age. In younger patients, regional metastases do not place patients at higher risk of disease-specific death. This young patient group has a higher rate of subsequent regional failure, but such recurrences can be detected early and cured with appropriate surgery. In contrast, older patients with regional disease at presentation are at a higher risk of death. These patients have higher rates of distant recurrence, which impacts on survival.

Distant metastases are uncommon.[19] In older patients, distant disease portends a grave prognosis. These patients cannot be cured surgically, and at advanced age, the response to radioactive iodine is limited, rendering the outcomes of treatment of systemic disease poor. In contrast, younger patients, particularly children, commonly present with pulmonary metastases. These young patients with extremely well differentiated cancers have iodine avid disease, which allows for excellent outcomes following adjuvant radioactive iodine (RAI) even in the presence of distant metastases.[19]

Following preoperative assessment, patients can be stratified into low-, intermediate- or high-risk groups based on host and tumor characteristics. Low-risk patients are young (<45 years) with low-risk tumors (pT1/2 N0 M0). High-risk cases are older (>45 years) with high-risk tumors (T3/4 or M1). The remaining young patients with high-risk disease and older patients with low-risk disease constitute an intermediate-risk group (**Table 1**).[20] Such an approach allows patients to be stratified for treatment based on risk versus benefit assessment. More recently, recurrence risk stratification systems have been developed that include variables such as the presence of nodal disease and the degree of ETE (**Table 2**).[17]

CLINICAL PRESENTATION/EXAMINATION

Most patients who present for thyroid surgery will have no signs or symptoms. However, this does not render clinical history and examination without clinical utility. The surgeon should elicit relevant features from the patient such as family history and exposure to ionizing radiation. The presence of high-risk features such as prior external beam radiation to the head and neck places the thyroid gland at higher risk of malignant change, and strengthens the case for total thyroidectomy. More significant symptoms such as voice change, dysphagia and hemoptysis suggest advanced disease.

Physical examination should include assessment of the general state of the patient, examination of the central neck and regional nodes, and assessment of vocal cord mobility in all patients. In those patients with a suspicion of fixation of the primary tumor, nodal metastases or vocal cord palsy, cross-sectional imaging of the head and neck, including the mediastinum, allows for an accurate assessment of disease extent.

In those patients considered to have invasive disease affecting the airway or esophagus, preoperative endoscopic assessment is essential to confirm the extent of disease and plan surgical therapy.

Table 1
Memorial Sloan Kettering Cancer Center cause-specific mortality risk classification system (GAMES)

Risk Level	Patient Factor	Tumor Factor			
Low risk	Age <45 y	Papillary Ca	M_0	No ETE	Size <4 cm
High risk	Age >45 y	Follicular Ca/Hurthle Cell Ca	M1	ETE	Size >4 cm
Low-risk case	Low-risk patient	Low-risk tumor			
Intermediate-risk case	Low-risk patient High-risk patient	High-risk tumor Low-risk tumor			
High-risk case	High-risk patient	High-risk tumor			

Table 2
American Thyroid Association risk of recurrence stratification

	Regional Metastases	Distant Metastases	Extrathyroid Extension	Surgical Resection	Aggressive Pathology	RAI Uptake Outside Thyroid Bed
Low risk: Only if all the following are true	Absent	Absent	Absent	Complete	Absent	Absent
Intermediate risk or High risk: In any of the following are true	Present	Absent Present	Microscopic Macroscopic	Complete Incomplete	Present	Present

AVAILABLE PROCEDURES AND CHOICE OF PROCEDURE

Procedures such as nodulectomy and subtotal thyroidectomy no longer have a role in the management of WDTC. The minimum procedure that should be considered is extracapsular thyroid lobectomy when unilateral surgery is performed, and total thyroidectomy when bilateral surgery is required. The only exception to this is isolated, uninodular isthmic lesions that can safely be managed in selected low-risk patients using thyroid isthmusectomy, thereby avoiding entry to the tracheoesophageal grooves and minimizing the morbidity of surgery.[21]

When selecting an appropriate surgical procedure, the surgeon must consider 3 factors: the need for resection of lymph nodes, the need for bilateral surgery, and the anticipated need for postoperative radioactive iodine (**Fig. 1**).

PLANNING PRIMARY THYROID SURGERY

The extent of appropriate primary thyroid surgery will be dictated by the estimation of risk following preoperative assessment. For high-risk patients with locally, regionally, or distantly aggressive disease, total thyroidectomy will be the procedure of choice. This procedure should achieve removal of all thyroid tissue in the central compartment, leaving the patient free of gross disease. By removing the entire thyroid, such patients are rendered suitable for radioactive iodine treatment, which has a role in the management of such high-risk cases.

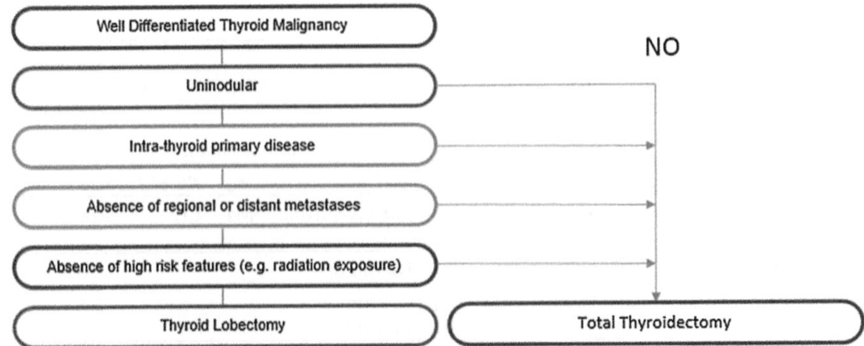

Fig. 1. Algorithm for selection of primary thyroid procedure.

In contrast, for younger patients (<45 years of age) with low-risk disease confined to the thyroid gland (cT1/2N0M0) and a sonographically normal contralateral lobe, thyroid lobectomy is sufficient to achieve cure and minimize recurrence rates, while protecting the contralateral recurrent nerve and parathyroid glands.[22–24] In this group, up to 90% of patients can be spared a contralateral lobectomy in the long term, thus achieving the goal of maximizing oncological outcome while minimizing morbidity.[22]

Those patients who are considered low risk, but have evidence of contralateral nodularity, present a challenge. Many will be adequately oncologically treated with unilateral surgery to resect the proven or suspected malignancy. However, contralateral nodules will not regress spontaneously, and will remain a source of anxiety for patient and clinician alike. Most of these patients are best served by total thyroidectomy to avoid the need for serial ultrasounds and needle aspirations, which in a young patient may be required for many years and are likely at some point to yield at least a suspicious result mandating further surgery. However, the threshold at which total thyroidectomy is performed in those situations is best determined by taking into account the overall health of the patients and their preference, instead of a single determinant such as the size of the nodule.

Occasionally patients will present with advanced local disease. Such patients require careful preoperative assessment. This complex group of patients will require assessment of the integrity of the recurrent nerves and involvement of the airway and gastrointestinal tract. The aim of surgery in this group is to remove all gross disease. Achieving this goal may require resection of vital structures within the central neck. In patients with superficial invasion of the airway framework, shave excision may suffice. Full-thickness involvement of the central neck viscera will require a through-and-through resection and reconstruction to restore function.[25] This heterogeneous group of patients requires a wide range of surgical procedures that are beyond the scope of this article but are covered elsewhere.[26,27]

PLANNING NECK DISSECTION

In terms of a surgical approach to planning the extent of required neck dissection, several preoperative factors should be considered:

- Evidence of metastasis to the lateral neck (yes/no)
- Evidence of metastasis to the central neck (yes/no)

In patients with evidence of metastasis to the lateral neck, therapeutic neck dissection should be planned. Regionally advanced thyroid cancer commonly involves levels II through V, and all levels should be comprehensively dissected in order to minimize the chance of persistent disease presenting at a later date.[28,29] These patients are considered at high risk of disease recurrence, and older patients are at higher risk of disease-related death. For this reason, most will be offered postoperative radioactive iodine, and therefore, total thyroidectomy will also be indicated.

In patients without evidence of lateral neck metastases should be managed conservatively. It is true that around 25% of cN0 patients will have occult disease in the lateral neck.[15] However, such disease rarely presents clinically, and the morbidity of lateral neck dissection is such that most experts do not recommend elective lateral neck dissection.[29]

Planning the approach to the central neck is more controversial. Those patients who have evidence of disease require a therapeutic dissection that resects all disease while preserving the recurrent nerve and parathyroid glands. Again, most such patients will be considered for radioactive iodine, and therefore total thyroidectomy will be preferred in such patients. It is true that some patients with limited, small volume regional metastases may be managed without radioactive iodine; however, the majority should be offered total thyroidectomy.

Those patients without overt evidence of central nodal metastases provide the controversy. Some groups advocate elective central neck dissection in such patients, as occult disease is encountered in up to 40% of these patients.[15] Particularly in the older group, this upstages patients to stage III, thereby justifying the use of radioactive iodine in groups following this philosophy. There is also some evidence that elective central neck surgery may lower postoperative thyroglobulin (Tg) levels.[30] In contrast, opponents highlight the fact that no group has ever demonstrated a survival advantage in those patients who are considered cN0. In addition, there is strong evidence that patients who have a central neck dissection are at higher risk of postoperative hypocalcemia and recurrent nerve injury.[31] In terms of lowering Tg levels, longer-term data have questioned the duration of this biochemical response.[32] A further argument against elective central neck dissection is the report of salvage neck surgery series. Clayman and colleagues[33] reported high levels of recurrent disease in areas not routinely addressed in elective surgery, such as dorsal to the recurrent nerve. Indeed there is growing evidence that a policy of observation of the cN0 central neck is safe in both the short and long terms, with low recurrence rates and excellent survival.[34] The concept of identifying subclinical disease in order to upstage such low-risk patients and inform them that their risk of death is elevated as a result is flawed.

Although the controversy over this issue is far from resolved, international guidelines are now moving away from recommending elective central neck surgery as routine in most cases to advocating a more selective approach to avoid treatment-related medical and surgical complications.[17]

DIAGNOSIS IN THE OPERATING ROOM

Following agreement between the patient, surgeon, and the endocrinologist, the operation can proceed. At this stage, the surgeon will be responsible not only for carrying out the agreed procedure, but also for evaluation of the findings in the operating room and acting accordingly.

Although advances in preoperative investigation have improved surgeons' ability to assess the burden of primary, regional, and distant disease, the surgeon must still be aware that findings in the operating room may mandate changes in surgical plan.

The aim of surgery is to resect all gross disease with clear margins, but also to avoid the need for further surgery. Not only must the surgeon consider the preoperative cytology and ultrasound features, he or she must also bear in mind the gross extent of disease, intraoperative frozen section results, and the risk status of the patient. With such an approach, the need for completion thyroidectomy can be minimized.

In patients who have indeterminate diagnosis of malignancy and undergo diagnostic lobectomy, the finding of regional metastases or ETE of primary disease confirms malignancy, which may mandate total thyroidectomy. In such cases, frozen section analysis of excised tissue can be used to confirm the diagnosis and justify a more aggressive surgical approach. In the event that frozen section analysis is equivocal, it is important that the patient understands that the surgeon will make a decision based upon all available factors in order to achieve the aims set out earlier, undertake the best oncologic procedure, and avoid completion thyroidectomy.

In those patients who are found to have intrathyroid disease, frozen section is of less clinical utility, as most patients have a report of "follicular lesion defer to permanent histology."[35] It is for this group of patients that the surgeon's integration of diagnostic

Table 3
Survival outcomes for patients with WDTC

Group	Risk Stratification System		10 y Survival (%)
Memorial Sloan Kettering Cancer Center	GAMES	Low	100
		Intermediate	98
		High	87
Mayo Clinic	MACIS	Low	100
		High	88
National Thyroid Cancer Treatment Cooperative Study Registry Group	AJCC staging	Stage I+II	100
		Stage III	90
		Stage IV	60

Abbreviations: AJCC, American Joint Committee on Cancer; GAMES, Grade, Age, Metastases, Extra-thyroid Extension, Size; MACIS, Metastasis, Age at presentation, Completness of surgical resection, Invasion (extrathyroidal), Size.

variables is most important. Such patients should be managed in a way such as to minimize the need for completion thyroidectomy.[36]

In contrast to disappointing results from intraoperative frozen section in this setting, the technique of frozen section can reliably be used to identify thyroid tissue in regional lymph nodes, and in order to confirm a suspected parathyroid gland encountered during dissection.

CLINICAL OUTCOMES IN THE LITERATURE

Patients with WDTC have excellent outcomes. Analysis of survival requires long-term follow-up and large cohorts. Several institutional studies and national database analyses have confirmed that survival of over 90% can be expected for the cohort as a whole. Low-risk patients, particularly those with intra-glandular disease, rarely die of disease. This group has survival outcomes that exceed 98% at 10 years, which should be borne in mind when planning potentially morbid treatment. In contrast, there remain patients who will have poorer outcomes, particularly older patients with advanced disease who need appropriate aggressive treatment. The results of major North American series are shown in **Table 3**.[1,8,37]

SUMMARY

Patients with WDTC have excellent outcomes when treated appropriately. An understanding of the biology of this increasingly common disease is important to allow clinicians to select appropriate therapy for their patients.

Surgeons should plan treatment following adequate preoperative investigation and in conjunction with the patient and the endocrinologist. Findings in the operating room may mandate changes to the operative plan, and the surgeon should be prepared to modify his or her approach accordingly.

In low-risk patients with intrathyroid disease, thyroid lobectomy results in cure for the vast majority of patients while minimizing the impact of surgery. For high-risk patients who are likely to require postoperative RAI, resection of the contralateral lobe facilitates adjuvant therapy. There is no role for elective lateral neck surgery, and enthusiasm for elective central neck surgery is waning, as oncological results have been disappointing while increased morbidity is evident. For those patients with nodal metastases, a compartment-orientated systematic neck dissection of levels II to V to remove all gross disease is required.

With appropriate treatment, survival outcomes are excellent, with almost no deaths expected from low-risk disease and over half of those considered high risk being alive at 10 years. There has been little improvement in outcomes for these selected high-risk patients. These patients should be the focus of the health care resources that will be increasingly expended given the rising incidence of thyroid cancer. Surgeons' efforts must not be consumed with more aggressive treatment for low-risk patients who do well irrespective of therapy, but with those patients who have worse outcomes and more to gain from intensification of therapy.

REFERENCES

1. Nixon IJ, Ganly I, Patel SG, et al. Changing trends in well differentiated thyroid carcinoma over eight decades. Int J Surg 2012;10:618–23.
2. Olaleye O, Ekrikpo U, Moorthy R, et al. Increasing incidence of differentiated thyroid cancer in South East England: 1987-2006. Eur Arch Otorhinolaryngol 2011; 268(6):899–906.
3. Davies L, Welch HG. Thyroid cancer survival in the United States: observational data from 1973 to 2005. Arch Otolaryngol Head Neck Surg 2010;136(5):440–4.
4. Solares CA, Penalonzo MA, Xu M, et al. Occult papillary thyroid carcinoma in postmortem species: prevalence at autopsy. Am J Otolaryngol 2005;26(2):87–90.
5. Harach HR, Franssila KO, Wasenius VM. Occult papillary carcinoma of the thyroid. A "normal" finding in Finland. A systematic autopsy study. Cancer 1985; 56(3):531–8.
6. Berge T, Lundberg S. Cancer in Malmo 1958-1969. An autopsy study. Acta Pathol Microbiol Scand Suppl 1977;(260):1–235.
7. Hughes DT, Haymart MR, Miller BS, et al. The most commonly occurring papillary thyroid cancer in the United States is now a microcarcinoma in a patient older than 45 years. Thyroid 2011;21(3):231–6.
8. Hay ID, Thompson GB, Grant CS, et al. Papillary thyroid carcinoma managed at the Mayo Clinic during six decades (1940-1999): temporal trends in initial therapy and long-term outcome in 2444 consecutively treated patients. World J Surg 2002;26(8):879–85.
9. Shaha AR, Shah JP, Loree TR. Risk group stratification and prognostic factors in papillary carcinoma of thyroid. Ann Surg Oncol 1996;3(6):534–8.
10. Cady B, Rossi R. An expanded view of risk-group definition in differentiated thyroid carcinoma. Surgery 1988;104(6):947–53.
11. Byar DP, Green SB, Dor P, et al. A prognostic index for thyroid carcinoma. A study of the E.O.R.T.C. Thyroid Cancer Cooperative Group. Eur J Cancer 1979;15(8): 1033–41.
12. Hay ID, Bergstralh EJ, Goellner JR, et al. Predicting outcome in papillary thyroid carcinoma: development of a reliable prognostic scoring system in a cohort of 1779 patients surgically treated at one institution during 1940 through 1989. Surgery 1993;114(6):1050–7 [discussion: 1057–8].
13. Edge SB, American Joint Committee on Cancer. AJCC cancer staging manual. 7th edition. New York: Springer; 2010. p. 648, xiv.
14. Riss JC, Peyrottes I, Chamorey E, et al. Prognostic impact of tumour multifocality in thyroid papillary microcarcinoma based on a series of 160 cases. Eur Ann Otorhinolaryngol Head Neck Dis 2012;129(4):175–8.
15. Hartl DM, Leboulleux S, Al Ghuzlan A, et al. Optimization of staging of the neck with prophylactic central and lateral neck dissection for papillary thyroid carcinoma. Ann Surg 2012;255(4):777–83.

16. Nixon IJ, Ganly I, Patel S, et al. The impact of microscopic extrathyroid extension on outcome in patients with clinical T1 and T2 well-differentiated thyroid cancer. Surgery 2011;150(6):1242–9.
17. Cooper DS, Doherty GM, Haugen BR, et al. Revised American Thyroid Association management guidelines for patients with thyroid nodules and differentiated thyroid cancer. Thyroid 2009;19(11):1167–214.
18. Mulla MG, Knoefel WT, Gilbert J, et al. Lateral cervical lymph node metastases in papillary thyroid cancer: a systematic review of imaging-guided and prophylactic removal of the lateral compartment. Clin Endocrinol (Oxf) 2012;77(1):126–31.
19. Nixon IJ, Whitcher M, Palmer FL, et al. The impact of distant metastases at presentation on prognosis in patients differentiated carcinoma of the thyroid gland. Thyroid 2012;22:884–9.
20. Shah JP, Loree TR, Dharker D, et al. Prognostic factors in differentiated carcinoma of the thyroid gland. Am J Surg 1992;164(6):658–61.
21. Nixon IJ, Palmer FL, Whitcher MM, et al. Thyroid isthmusectomy for well-differentiated thyroid cancer. Ann Surg Oncol 2011;18(3):767–70.
22. Nixon IJ, Ganly I, Patel SG, et al. Thyroid lobectomy for treatment of well differentiated intrathyroid malignancy. Surgery 2012;151(4):571–9.
23. Vaisman F, Shaha A, Fish S, et al. Initial therapy with either thyroid lobectomy or total thyroidectomy without radioactive iodine remnant ablation is associated with very low rates of structural disease recurrence in properly selected patients with differentiated thyroid cancer. Clin Endocrinol (Oxf) 2011;75:112–9.
24. Barney BM, Hitchcock YJ, Sharma P, et al. Overall and cause-specific survival for patients undergoing lobectomy, near-total, or total thyroidectomy for differentiated thyroid cancer. Head Neck 2011;33(5):645–9.
25. McCaffrey JC. Aerodigestive tract invasion by well-differentiated thyroid carcinoma: diagnosis, management, prognosis, and biology. Laryngoscope 2006; 116(1):1–11.
26. Nixon IJ, Ganly I, Shah JP. Thyroid cancer: surgery for the primary tumor. Oral Oncol 2013;49(7):654–8.
27. Price DL, Wong RJ, Randolph GW. Invasive thyroid cancer: management of the trachea and esophagus. Otolaryngol Clin North Am 2008;41(6):1155–68, ix–x.
28. Wu G, Fraser S, Pai SI, et al. Determining the extent of lateral neck dissection necessary to establish regional disease control and avoid reoperation after previous total thyroidectomy and radioactive iodine for papillary thyroid cancer. Head Neck 2012;34(10):1418–21.
29. Ferris R, Goldenberg D, Haymart MR, et al. American Thyroid Association consensus review of the anatomy, terminology and rationale for lateral neck dissection in differentiated thyroid cancer. Thyroid 2012;22(5):501–8.
30. Sywak M, Cornford L, Roach P, et al. Routine ipsilateral level VI lymphadenectomy reduces postoperative thyroglobulin levels in papillary thyroid cancer. Surgery 2006;140(6):1000–5 [discussion: 1005–7].
31. Giordano D, Valcavi R, Thompson GB, et al. Complications of central neck dissection in patients with papillary thyroid carcinoma: results of a study on 1087 patients and review of the literature. Thyroid 2012;22(9):911–7.
32. Popadich A, Levin O, Lee JC, et al. A multicenter cohort study of total thyroidectomy and routine central lymph node dissection for cN0 papillary thyroid cancer. Surgery 2011;150(6):1048–57.
33. Clayman GL, Agarwal G, Edeiken BS, et al. Long-term outcome of comprehensive central compartment dissection in patients with recurrent/persistent papillary thyroid carcinoma. Thyroid 2011;21(12):1309–16.

34. Monchik JM, Simon CJ, Caragacianu DL, et al. Does failure to perform prophylactic level VI node dissection leave persistent disease detectable by ultrasonography in patients with low-risk papillary carcinoma of the thyroid? Surgery 2009; 146(6):1182–7.
35. Rosario PW, Reis JS, Padrao EL, et al. The utility of frozen section evaluation for follicular thyroid lesions. Ann Surg Oncol 2004;11(9):879.
36. Shaha AR, Jaffe BM. Completion thyroidectomy: a critical appraisal. Surgery 1992;112(6):1148–52 [discussion: 1152–3].
37. Sherman SI, Brierley JD, Sperling M, et al. Prospective multicenter study of thyroiscarcinoma treatment: initial analysis of staging and outcome. National Thyroid Cancer Treatment Cooperative Study Registry Group. Cancer 1998;83(5):1012–21.

Contemporary Surgical Techniques

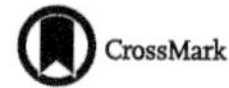

William S. Duke, MD, Katrina Chaung, MD, David J. Terris, MD*

KEYWORDS

- Thyroid surgery • Thyroid cancer • Endoscopic • Robotic • Minimally invasive

KEY POINTS

- Two divergent paradigms have developed for reducing the cosmetic burden of thyroid surgery: minimally invasive anterior cervical approaches and remote access approaches.
- Minimally invasive cervical approaches use small incisions on the anterior neck for direct access to the thyroid compartment and require limited dissection to remove the thyroid gland.
- Remote access approaches use well-hidden incisions but should not be considered minimally invasive, given the increased extent of dissection required and the resultant prolonged recovery compared with that of minimally invasive anterior cervical approaches.
- These alternative approaches have been applied to small, low-risk, well-differentiated thyroid cancers with promising and oncologically appropriate results. Careful patient selection and comprehensive preoperative counseling is essential.

INTRODUCTION

Conventional thyroidectomy techniques, although appropriate in some cases, yield a conspicuous anterior cervical scar that may be difficult to camouflage. Patient-driven motivations to decrease the cosmetic impact of thyroid procedures have generated procedures that aim to minimize the visible scar and improve postoperative recovery. Two distinct pathways have emerged from these efforts. One track created minimally invasive anterior cervical approaches that strive to decrease the incisional length and extent of dissection while providing direct and anatomically familiar access to the thyroid gland. The other developed remote access techniques that approach the thyroid gland from extracervical vantage points using endoscopic and robotic assistance, consequently removing the thyroidectomy scar from the visible neck. For the appropriate patients, these are viable techniques that accomplish both the surgical and cosmetic goals. The role of these procedures in treating malignant thyroid disease has been recently evaluated.

Disclosures: Dr W.S. Duke, Dr K. Chaung: None; Dr D.J. Terris: Directed thyroid courses sponsored by Johnson & Johnson.
Department of Otolaryngology, Georgia Regents University, 1120 Fifteenth Street, BP-4109, Augusta, GA 30912-4060, USA
* Corresponding author.
E-mail address: dterris@gru.edu

Otolaryngol Clin N Am 47 (2014) 529–544
http://dx.doi.org/10.1016/j.otc.2014.04.002
0030-6665/14/$ – see front matter

BACKGROUND AND HISTORY

In the late 1800s, Emil Theodor Kocher revolutionized the field of thyroid surgery, transforming the thyroidectomy from a perilous operation with sometimes dire consequences to a validated and accepted procedure. For more than a century, his traditional method, which involved a large 7- to 10-cm transverse cervical incision, elevation of subplatysmal flaps, and routine postoperative drainage and inpatient care, was routinely performed.[1] The development and widespread utilization of endoscopic and minimally invasive techniques in other surgical fields provoked interest in their application to neck surgery. In 1996, Gagner[2] described the first endoscopic cervical surgery, using multiple ports and CO_2 insufflation to perform a subtotal parathyroidectomy. Although the cosmetic outcome was ostensibly excellent, the procedure took 5 hours, produced mild hypercarbia and significant subcutaneous emphysema, and necessitated a 4-day inpatient admission.[3] This experience, while demonstrating issues that would need to be overcome before these techniques could be widely used, elicited the attention of patients and surgeons to the possibility of alternative approaches to the thyroid compartment.

These alternative approaches developed along 2 avenues: minimally invasive and remote access approaches (**Table 1**). Along the minimally invasive anterior cervical pathway, both minimally invasive video-assisted thyroidectomy (MIVAT)[4,5] and minimally invasive nonendoscopic thyroidectomy (MINET)[6] were cultivated. These approaches camouflage incisions that are significantly smaller than those of a conventional thyroidectomy in natural neck creases and reduce the extent of dissection, obviating postoperative drainage and reducing postoperative pain. Not only is the cosmetic impact reduced but also outpatient surgery becomes feasible with these techniques.[7] The other pathway pursued remote access approaches that primarily emerged in Asian practices, tailored to a population at increased risk of hypertrophic scarring and highly cognizant of postoperative cosmesis.[8,9] Although not completely scarless, these techniques eliminate any scar from the visible neck by accessing the thyroid compartment by way of a more distant but concealed site. Consequently, more extensive dissection is required and anatomic structures not otherwise

Table 1
Alternative approaches to the thyroid compartment

Approach	Incision Site	Technique
Minimally invasive anterior cervical	Anterior neck	1. MIVAT 2. MINET
Remote access	Chest or breast	1. CO_2 assisted • Endoscopic 2. Gasless • Endoscopic • Robotic
	Axillary	1. CO_2 assisted • Endoscopic 2. Gasless • Endoscopic • RAT
	Combined	1. ABBA 2. BABA • Endoscopic • Robotic
	Postauricular	1. RFT

encountered during a traditional thyroidectomy are placed at risk of injury. Additionally, some techniques require postoperative drainage and hospital admission.

As with Gagner group's[3] initial endoscopic experience, early efforts with these alternative approaches used endoscopic visualization and were contingent on CO_2 insufflation to maintain an adequate operative pocket.[4,10–12] Given the previously mentioned drawbacks associated with CO_2 insufflation,[13] gasless techniques were explored. The minimally invasive anterior cervical approaches use blunt retraction of soft tissue[5,14] and some remote access techniques use percutaneous suspension techniques[15–17] or specialized retractors[18] to render CO_2 insufflation unnecessary to maintain the operative space. Although these modifications were conducive to performing cosmetically conscious thyroid surgery, concerns remained regarding the ability to perform oncologically sound surgeries with these alternative approaches.

ADVANTAGES AND DISADVANTAGES OF ALTERNATIVE APPROACHES

Long-term morbidity and mortality after traditional thyroid surgery are rare[19,20] and may potentially be even lower in minimally invasive video-assisted anterior cervical approaches.[21,22] When performed by experienced surgeons, MIVAT and MINET techniques can lead to shorter operative times, less blood loss, less postoperative pain, and improved cosmetic outcomes compared with conventional thyroid surgery, while still providing an anatomically familiar route of access.[21,23] Bilateral resection can also be performed without necessitating an additional scar.[14]

Although minimally invasive, MIVAT and MINET generate a small but visible anterior neck scar. An assistant to operate the endoscope is also necessary in the MIVAT technique. Not all patients who require thyroid surgery are appropriate for MINET and MIVAT, because the minimally invasive approach may be difficult or even unsafe in instances of large goiters, substernal or retropharyngeal extension, or thyroiditis. Furthermore, patients with thyroid malignancies need to be carefully considered to provide the most oncologically appropriate surgery for their disease.

Remote access procedures provide an attractive alternative for individuals who find any visible cervical scar an unacceptable outcome. The various access sites and more extensive dissection required make it difficult to directly compare the degree of postoperative pain or length of recovery for this group as a whole to traditional thyroid surgery.[24–26] The increased dissection and unconventional anatomic view of the thyroid compartment may also affect surgical times, although this is highly dependent on surgeon experience and technique.[25–27] The increased medical resource expenditure associated with remote access surgery versus traditional thyroid surgery has been demonstrated.[24,28–30]

There is concern over obtaining enough exposure and visualization in these alternative approaches to adequately remove thyroid tissue and, if indicated, perform a nodal dissection in cases of malignancies to ensure a reliable oncological outcome. To address these concerns, the suitability of both minimally invasive and some remote access techniques in treating thyroid cancers has been evaluated.

APPROACHES

Minimally Invasive Anterior Cervical

Minimally invasive video-assisted thyroidectomy

- Prior to surgery, a 15- to 20-mm cervical incision is marked in a low natural skin crease with the patient awake and upright to ensure a vertically favorable position in the neck.

- The incision is carried through the platysma until the sternohyoid and sternothyroid muscles are encountered.
- No subplatysmal flaps are elevated.
- The strap muscles are separated vertically in the midline, bluntly dissected off the anterior and lateral aspect of the thyroid gland, and retracted laterally.
- Under visualization with a 5-mm 30° laparoscope, the avascular space between the inferior constrictor muscle and the medial aspect of the superior pole is bluntly dissected, isolating the superior vascular pedicle.
- The superior pole vessels are divided close to the thyroid capsule with Harmonic ACE shears, ACE23P (Ethicon Endo-Surgery, Cincinnati, Ohio) (**Fig. 1**). Care is taken to identify and preserve the superior parathyroid gland.
- The middle thyroid vein is then isolated and divided, allowing mobilization of the inferior pole. The inferior pole vessels are divided, with care taken to identify and preserve the inferior parathyroid gland.
- The lobe is exteriorized with gentle traction using hemostat clamps placed directly on the gland, especially the superior pole. Once delivered externally, the lobe is retracted medially and ventrally and the recurrent laryngeal nerve (RLN) identified (**Fig. 2**).
- The nerve is carefully traced until it courses under the inferior constrictor muscle.
- If only a lobectomy is performed, the isthmus is divided and the lobe delivered from the field. If a total thyroidectomy is indicated, the contralateral lobe is removed in a similar manner.
- The surgical field is irrigated with saline and Surgicel (Ethicon, Somerville, New Jersey) is placed into the thyroid bed.
- The strap muscles are reapproximated in the midline with a single 3-0 Vicryl suture (Ethicon) in a figure-of-8 configuration. This single fixation point decreases the risk of postoperative airway obstruction by allowing any fluid accumulation to egress from the thyroid compartment.
- The subcutaneous tissues are closed with buried interrupted 4-0 Vicryl sutures, the superficial skin layer reapproximated with tissue adhesive and a single $^{1}/_{4}$ inch Steri-Strip (3M, St. Paul, Minnesota) is placed over the incision (**Fig. 3**). The procedure is performed on an outpatient basis without postoperative drainage.

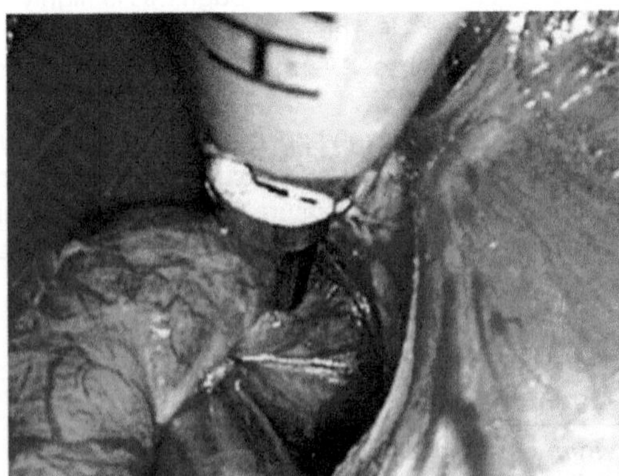

Fig. 1. Bundle ligation of the superior vascular pedicle with an advanced energy device during MIVAT. (*From* Terris DJ, Seybt MW. Modifications of Miccoli minimally invasive thyroidectomy for the low-volume surgeon. Am J Otolaryngol 2011;32:395; with permission.)

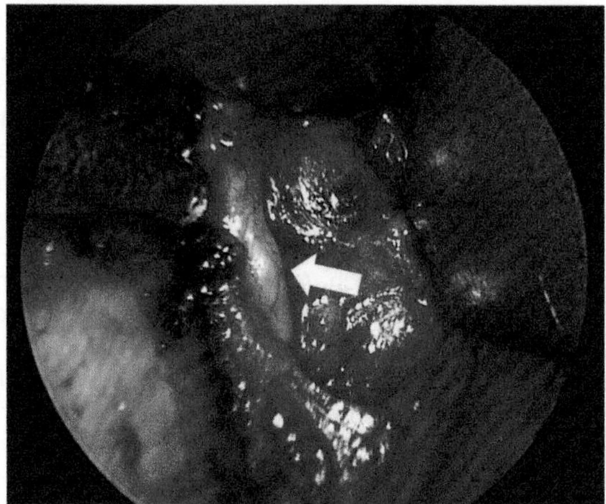

Fig. 2. Identification of the RLN (*arrow*) is facilitated by the magnified endoscopic view available during an MIVAT.

Patient selection Initially considered for only small-volume benign lesions, patient selection criteria have expanded to include nodule size as large as 35 mm, estimated thyroid volume less than 25 cm^3, absence of thyroiditis, and no history of previous neck surgery or irradiaton. Some investigators have reported criteria that include thyroiditis, cytologically indeterminate nodules, and low- and even intermediate-risk differentiated thyroid cancers (DTCs), according to American Thyroid Association staging, that are less than 20 mm.[14,31,32] Reported contraindications have included nodules larger than 35 mm, estimated thyroid volume greater than 25 cm^3, severe thyroiditis, malignancies larger than 20 mm, and the presence or suspicion of nodal metastases.[31]

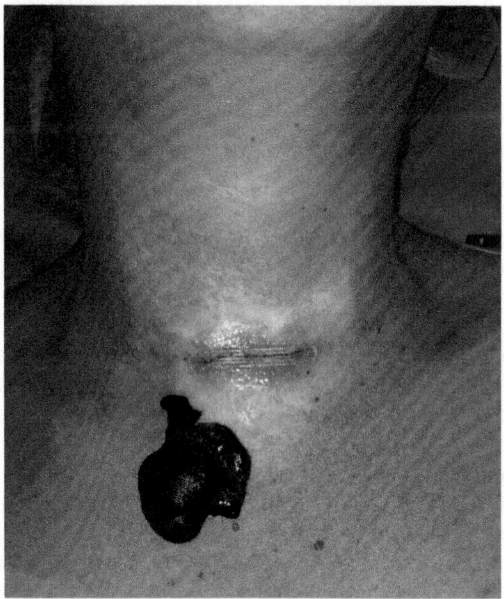

Fig. 3. The MIVAT incision is closed with tissue adhesive and a $\frac{1}{4}$ inch sterile strip.

An early multi-institutional trial that included 336 patients demonstrated a mean operative time of 69.4 minutes for a hemithyroidectomy and 87.4 minutes for total thyroidectomy with MIVAT. Complications included hemorrhage in 0.9% of cases, temporary RLN weakness in 2.1% of cases, permanent RLN weakness in 0.3% of cases, a temporary hypocalcemia rate of 2.7%, permanent hypocalcemia in 0.6% of patients, and a conversion rate of 4.5%.[33,34] This safety profile was corroborated in a large North American study of 228 patients.[22] Terris and Seybt[35] described several important modifications (detailed previously) designed to aid with MIVAT procedures as well as any anterior cervical approach. An important limitation is the obligate need for 2 surgical assistants: 1 to maintain the operative field with retractors and 1 to maneuver the endoscope.

The oncologic soundness of MIVAT thyroid cancers has been evaluated.[31,34] Miccoli and colleagues[34] described a series in which 33 patients with biopsy-proven low-risk (T1) papillary carcinomas were randomized to either MIVAT or conventional total thyroidectomy. To measure the completeness of resection, serum thyroglobulin levels and iodine 131 uptake scans were obtained 1 month postoperatively, with no significant difference found between the 2 groups. Although there were 3 cases of transient RLN palsy and 1 case of permanent hypoparathyroidism, there was no significant difference in the frequency of these complications between the 2 groups.

The prevalence of occult lymph node metastasis in DTC in the central compartment has been reported at 50% to 60%.[32] Debate continues regarding the benefit of elective neck dissection in low-risk DTC patients. Some investigators argue a possible survival benefit and reduced risk of nodal recurrence whereas others argue the potential risk to the RLN and parathyroid glands outweigh the benefits. Neidich and Steward[32] retrospectively assessed outcomes in cases of total or completion thyroidectomy and elective central neck dissection by MIVAT. Dissection of prelaryngeal, pretracheal, and either unilateral or bilateral paratracheal nodal basins was performed with a mean yield of 5.2 lymph nodes per patient; 11 of 28 patients harbored central compartment lymph nodes positive for metastases on pathology. The majority of the final pathology was consistent with papillary thyroid cancer; the remaining diagnoses included follicular and medullary carcinoma. Fifteen patients underwent radioiodine ablation. No recurrences were recorded during a median follow-up period of 14 months; 91% of the patients had low or undetectable thyroglobulin levels, defined as less than 1 ng/mL, and the remaining 2 patients had levels less than 1.5 ng/mL. No instances of permanent hypocalcemia or RLN palsy occurred. The reported rate of conversion to open surgery is rare but has been described for reasons, including early surgeon experience, difficult dissection, excessive bleeding, and preoperatively understaged cancer, where local tumor infiltration or metastatic lymph nodes were identified intraoperatively.[14,31] Thus, the possibility of extension to a conventional incision must be discussed with patients preoperatively.

Promising oncologic outcomes, as evidenced by postoperative serum thyroglobulin levels and radioiodine scintigraphy results comparable to those obtained after conventional thyroidectomies, support the viability of MIVAT for low-risk DTC.[14,32,33]

Minimally invasive nonendoscopic thyroidectomy

Almost concurrently with the development of MIVAT, groups in South Korea[23] and the United States[36] reported a minimally invasive nonendoscopic thyroidectomy (MINET) approach. This technique also strived to minimize incisional size and dissection extent compared with conventional thyroidectomy but without the addition of endoscopic instrumentation.

- Prior to surgery, a 3- to 5-cm cervical incision is marked in a low natural skin crease with the patient awake and upright to ensure a vertically favorable position in the neck.
- Dissection is performed in a similar fashion to that of the MIVAT approach.
- Without endoscopic magnification, positioning of retractors in a favorable vector maintains optimal exposure via the slightly longer incision through which both thyroidectomy and central neck dissection may be performed.[23]
- Closure is identical to the MIVAT technique and the patient is managed on an outpatient basis without postoperative drainage.

MINET has been demonstrated to be a safe and effective procedure in appropriately selected individuals. A retrospective comparison of patients undergoing MINET versus conventional thyroidectomy demonstrated MINET cases having a shorter operative time, less blood loss, a briefer hospital stay, decreased drain utilization, and less postoperative pain, with no significant difference in complication rates.[23] Limitations of MINET include inability to remove some large nodules or substernal goiters, in which case conventional thyroidectomy may be more appropriate. Oncologically, there is concern for the potential of missing positive lymph nodes, either in the contralateral tracheoesophageal groove due to inadequate visualization or in the lateral lymph node compartments if involved.[23]

In the same retrospective study,[23] central neck dissection was performed in more than 80% of the patients with malignancy in both the MINET and conventional thyroidectomy groups. There was no significant difference in either the number of central neck nodes dissected per patient or the number of positive lymph nodes identified per patient. In a prospective nonrandomized study by Cavicchi and colleagues,[37] MINET was performed on patients with papillary thyroid carcinoma; postoperative iodine 131 uptake was found to range from 0% to 2.13%. A completion thyroidectomy for malignancy on final pathology was also performed in 1 patient through the same incision. The cosmetic result was regarded as excellent in all patients. Selection criteria were similar to those for MIVAT.[23,36,37]

Remote Access Endoscopic

Chest/Breast approaches

In 2000, Ohgami and colleagues[10] described a series of CO_2 insufflation–assisted endoscopic hemithyroidectomies, which were considered the first truly remote access thyroidectomy procedures. Access was achieved through incisions at the parasternal border of 1 breast and along the superior margins of both areolas. Using a low insufflation pressure of 6 mm Hg, endoscopic dissection was conducted superiorly and superficially to the strap muscles to expose and remove the thyroid lobe.

Since that initial description, several variations of the anterior chest and breast approach have been described, including isolated anterior chest wall approaches[16] as well as bilateral[38] and unilateral[39] transareolar approaches. Recent studies reported indications, including unilateral benign lesions up to 3 cm that required removal to relieve compressive symptoms or cosmetic deformity and lesions positive for papillary carcinoma on cytology measuring less than 2 cm; patients must also not have suspicious or positive lymphadenopathy or a prior history of neck surgery or irradiation.[16,17,38,39] There is potential need to convert to a conventional approach should a central or lateral neck dissection be warranted[39]; however, in an early series, subtotal thyroidectomy and pretracheal and bilateral paratracheal lymph node dissections were performed without conversion to the conventional approach on patients with malignant tumors ranging from 1.0 to 2.3 cm.[16]

Although these approaches eliminate scars on the visible neck, they generate incisions on the anterior chest that are prone to hypertrophic scarring,[40] and on the breast, which may be an unappealing consideration for North American patients.[41,42] Additionally, these approaches have a narrow operative field, with restricted range of movement of the rigid endoscopic equipment.[40] These limitations prompted the development of other remote access techniques.

Axillary approaches

Ikeda and colleagues[11] described the endoscopic axillary approach, the first remote access alternative to the anterior chest and breast approach. In this technique, the patient is positioned supine on an operating table with the arm ipsilateral to the dissection elevated to expose the axilla. An axillary incision is made and dissection advances along the pectoralis major muscle until the platysma is encountered. Trocars are placed though the incision and CO_2 insufflation applied to maintain visualization of the operative field. Under endoscopic visualization, dissection continues between the anterior border of the sternocleidomastoid muscle (SCM) and the strap muscles until the thyroid lobe is encountered. The strap muscles are divided.

Although the cosmetic impact is less conspicuous compared with conventional surgery, this approach takes significantly longer to perform than a conventional open thyroidectomy.[43] The narrow operative field, reliance on rigid endoscopic instruments, and potential morbidity related to CO_2 insufflation are obvious limitations. Gasless remote access techniques that do not require a closed operative pocket and CO_2 insufflation were developed to overcome these drawbacks.[44] Later modifications of this approach involved dissection between the sternal and clavicular heads of the SCM rather than between the SCM and the sternohyoid muscles.[45]

This gasless technique has been described for thyroidectomy and central compartment node dissection of low-risk papillary thyroid carcinoma without need for open conversion. In 1 series of 410 malignant cases, no recurrences were observed in a follow-up range of 10 to 18 months, and thyroglobulin levels were less than 1 ng/mL in more than 90% of the cases; 71 patients underwent radioiodine ablation with subsequent iodine 131 scans, which showed no uptake. The investigators cited the advantage of approaching the thyroid bed between the SCM heads and dissecting along the anterior surface of the carotid sheath, allowing complete dissection of the ipsilateral central neck compartment, including both the prelaryngeal and paraesophageal lymph nodal packets.[45] Another report described successful unilateral lobectomy and isthmusectomy with central compartment dissection for papillary thyroid microcarcinoma using this approach.[44]

Several hybrid approaches, combining axillary and areolar incisions, were also developed. These techniques include the axillo-bilateral breast approach (ABBA)[40] and the bilateral axillo-breast approach (BABA).[46] These approaches exploit the cosmetic benefit of the axillary approaches while providing additional anterior chest working ports without producing a transverse parasternal scar (**Fig. 4**). Despite their cosmetic appeal, these approaches have been associated with several complications not typically associated with traditional thyroid surgery, including transient neuropraxia of the brachial plexus[47] and pneumothorax.[46]

Remote Access Robotic Procedures

The incorporation of da Vinci surgical robotic technology (Intuitive Surgical, Sunnyvale, California) in remote access thyroid surgery has granted surgeons a high-definition, 3-D view of the operative field while incorporating surgical instrumentation with a range of motion exceeding the capabilities of traditional rigid endoscopic

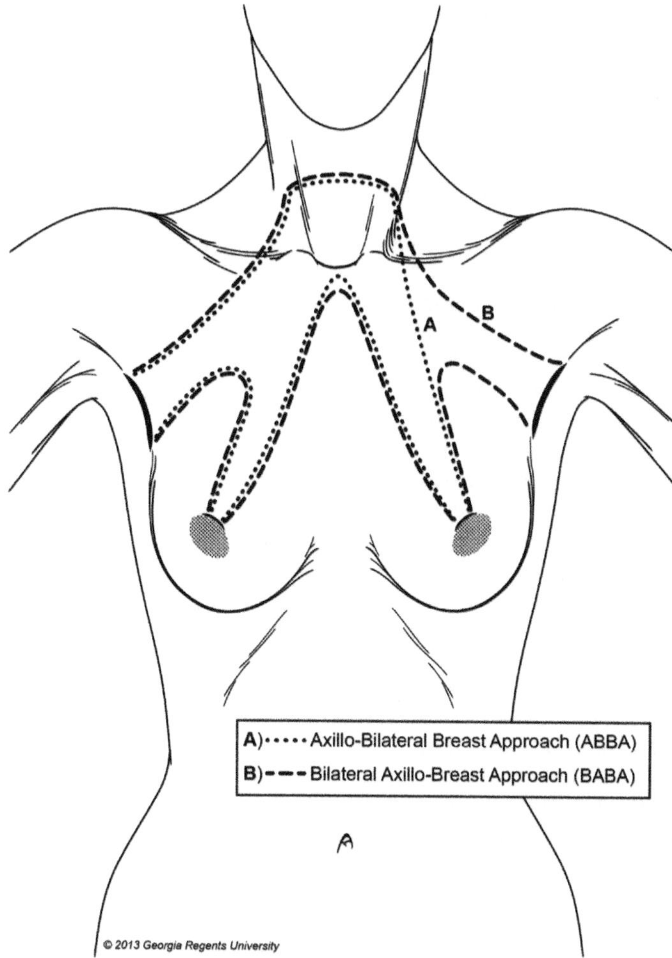

Fig. 4. Differences in the extent of dissection for the ABBA and the BABA. (*Courtesy of* Georgia Regents University; with permission.)

equipment. The first use of the surgical robot in thyroid surgery involved a combined robotic and endoscopic transaxillary approach with CO_2 insufflation to perform a thyroid lobectomy.[48] Robotic instrumentation has been incorporated into a CO_2-assisted BABA[49] and, more recently, a gasless dual-incision axillary and chest wall,[18] single incision axillary,[50] and facelift[51] approaches. This technology has also been used for central and lateral neck dissections for malignant disease.[52] Although Food and Drug Administration approval exists for robotic-assisted general surgery procedures, a specific indication for robotic thyroidectomy has not been issued.

Bilateral axillo-breast approach

A robotic BABA to perform total thyroidectomy and ipsilateral central neck dissection has been described for low-risk well-differentiated thyroid carcinoma with low postoperative thyroglobulin levels, reflecting the completeness of the resection. Complications rates were also comparable to conventional thyroidectomy techniques.[49] This technique, however, has not been embraced in North American practices.

Robotic axillary thyroidectomy

Completely robotic thyroid surgery was first reported in South Korea in 2009.[18,25,45] The robotic axillary thyroidectomy (RAT) permits a gasless dissection through an axillary portal. This was facilitated by inserting a specialized retractor (Chung [Marina Medical, Sunrise, Florida]) to elevate the skin and muscle flap for exposure.[45] Early descriptions also used a second parasternal incision on the anterior chest wall for a dual-incision approach,[25,45] but a single incision in the axilla[50] is now more commonly performed.

Kang and colleagues[25,45] described subtotal and total thyroidectomies with ipsilateral central neck dissection via RAT for papillary thyroid carcinomas less than 2 cm. Another series reported comparable surgical completeness and complication rates and improved cosmetic satisfaction after RAT compared with conventional approaches in patients with papillary thyroid cancer.[53] A multi-institutional study of low-risk papillary thyroid carcinoma patients undergoing RAT resection reported similar outcomes compared with those of patients undergoing conventional or endoscopic-assisted approaches.[27]

Early enthusiasm for this approach in the United States has subsided principally as a result of the emergence of several serious complications not previously experienced with conventional and other alternative approaches.[28,30,53–57]

Robotic facelift thyroidectomy

The complications encountered with the RAT experience in the United States along with the need for postoperative drains and inpatient care with this procedure prompted investigation into alternate avenues for robotic access to the thyroid compartment. The robotic facelift thyroidectomy (RFT) was developed in part to overcome the disadvantages associated with RAT (**Fig. 5**).[51,58]

The RFT incision begins in the postauricular crease and crosses into the occipital hairline (**Fig. 6**). A subplatysmal flap is elevated until the SCM is encountered. The great auricular nerve (GAN) and external jugular vein (EJV) are identified and preserved.

A muscular triangle bounded by the anterior border of the SCM, the superior border of the omohyoid muscle, and the posterior border of the sternohyoid is defined (**Fig. 7**). The omohyoid and other strap muscles are elevated ventrally, exposing the superior pole of the thyroid gland and the superior vascular pedicle. The surgical pocket is maintained with a modified Chung retractor to retract the strap muscles ventrally and a Singer hook (Medtronic, Jacksonville, Florida) to retract the SCM laterally and dorsally. The robot is deployed, using 3 arms with a 30° down-facing endoscope, a Harmonic device (Ethicon Endo-Surgery) in the dominant arm, and a Maryland grasper (Intuitive Surgical, Sunnyvale, California) in the nondominant arm.

The superior vascular pedicle is isolated and divided with the Harmonic device, allowing the superior thyroid pole to be retracted inferiorly and ventrally, exposing the inferior constrictor muscle. Care is taken to preserve the superior laryngeal nerve and superior parathyroid gland, which is reflected away from the posterior aspect of the thyroid gland. The RLN is then identified laterally just before it courses under the inferior constrictor (**Fig. 8**). The ligament of Berry is transected, the middle thyroid vein is divided, and the vessels of the inferior pole are ligated, taking care to preserve the inferior parathyroid gland. The isthmus is divided. Finally, remaining attachments between the thyroid lobe and the anterior trachea are divided and the specimen is removed. The wound is closed as previously described for the MIVAT procedure. RFT is performed on an outpatient basis and no postoperative drains are used.

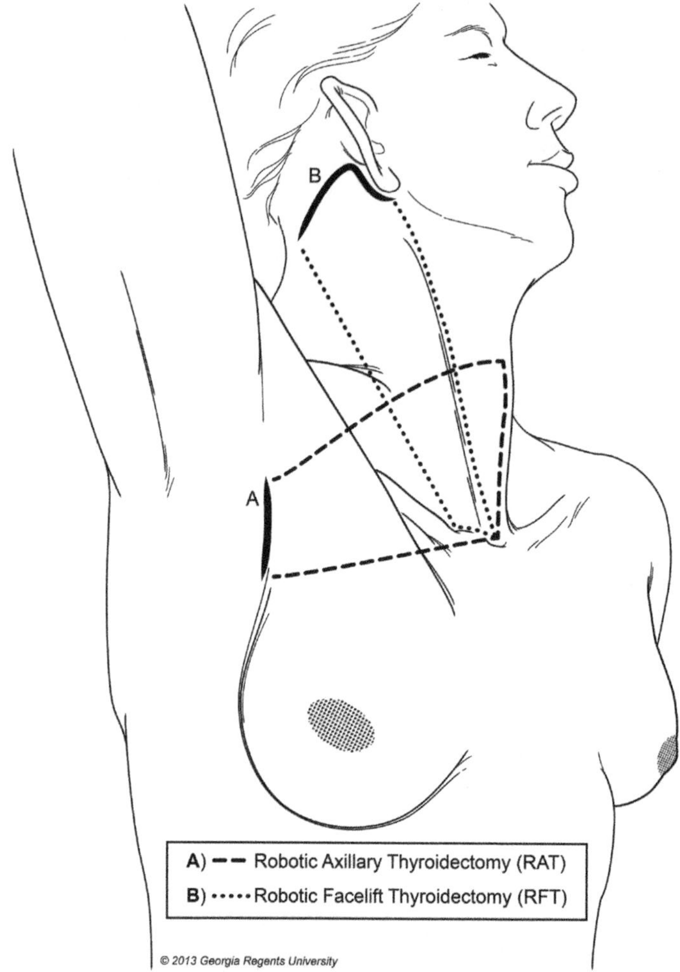

Fig. 5. Differences in the extent of dissection for the RFT and the RAT. (*Courtesy of* Georgia Regents University; with permission.)

Criteria for RFT eligibility include: dominant nodule size less than 4 cm, absence of clinically apparent thyroiditis, substernal extension, pathologic lymphadenopathy, or extrathyroidal disease and body mass index less than 40 kg/m^2.[59] Patients should be highly motivated to avoid a visible cervical scar and preoperative counseling should also be held regarding the unlikely risk of conversion to an anterior cervical approach. Overall health status should also be appropriate to tolerate the extended general anesthesia necessary to undergo this procedure (approximately 2 hours).[51]

In general, the thyroid disease to be addressed should be amenable to unilateral surgery because the approach vector and current instrumentation only permit unilateral surgery through a single ipsilateral incision. Staged bilateral completion thyroidectomy or total thyroidectomy RFT procedures, however, through 2 incisions have been reported for small, low-risk papillary thyroid carcinoma.[51]

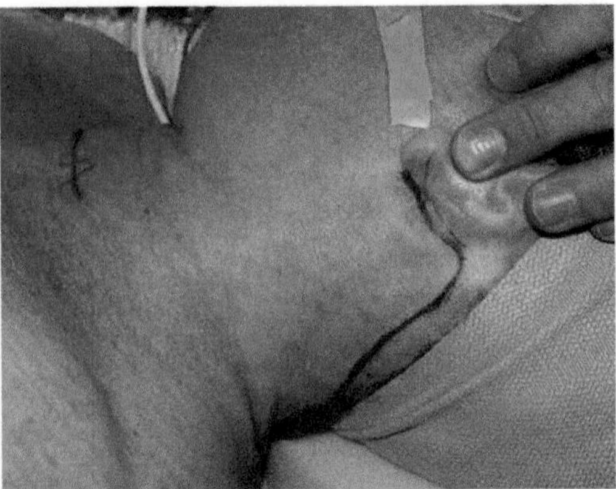

Fig. 6. RFT incision. (*From* Terris DJ, Singer MC, Seybt MW. Robotic facelift thyroidectomy: patient selection and technical considerations. Surg Laparosc Endosc Percutan Tech 2011;21:238; with permission.)

RFT is a recent option for remote access to the thyroid compartment. More than 60 procedures have been accomplished in the authors' center. In peer-reviewed publications, the procedures were completed on an outpatient basis without drainage in all but the first patient.[51,58,60] Complications rates have been low with 1 incidence of transient vocal fold weakness and 2 seromas, all of which resolved without intervention. There have been no instances of hypocalcemia or any conversions to an anterior cervical approach. This approach has been replicated in at least 4 other centers, amassing more than 100 cases that have been accomplished with similar safety profiles as described in the original reports.

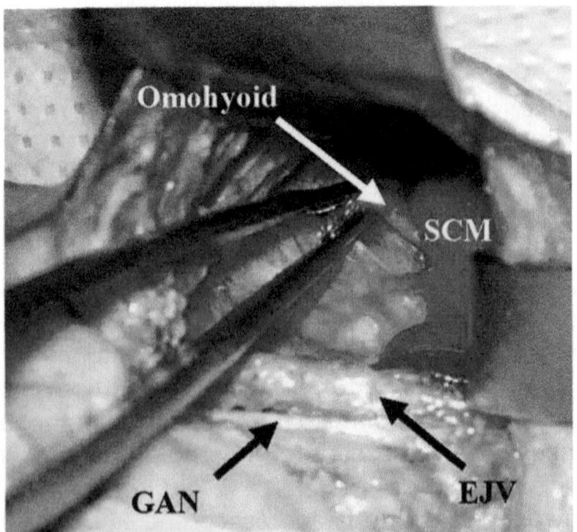

Fig. 7. The dissection pocket for a right-sided RFT. The GAN and EJV are preserved on the surface of the SCM. The SCM is retracted laterally, exposing the omohyoid and sternohyoid muscles. (*From* Terris DJ, Singer MC, Seybt MW. Robotic facelift thyroidectomy: II. Clinical feasibility and safety. Laryngoscope 2011;121:1638; with permission.)

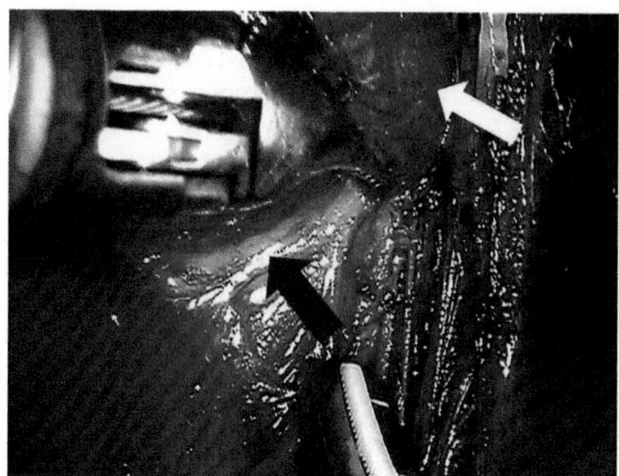

Fig. 8. The RLN (*black arrow*) is identified after retracting the thyroid gland (*white arrow*) ventrally during RFT.

SUMMARY

In response to patient-driven desires for improved cosmesis and personalized surgery, two distinct alternative approaches in thyroid surgery have been developed. Minimally invasive anterior cervical approaches aim to decrease both the incisional length and the extent of dissection, leading to an improved cosmetic outcome and postoperative experience, respectively. Remote access approaches exchange the scar from the visible anterior neck for a hidden scar but are associated with a greater extent of dissection and potential risk to anatomic structures not usually affected during other thyroid surgery approaches.

Although reports thus far have been encouraging regarding the oncologic soundness of some alternative approaches for small, low-risk, well-differentiated thyroid cancers, longer follow-up periods and greater experience may be needed before definite inclusional criteria for malignant disease are set. Preoperative discussion regarding the possibility of open conversion and reoperation is imperative.

Careful patient selection is paramount, and for the appropriate and committed patient, these innovative techniques provide a benefit not offered by conventional approaches.

REFERENCES

1. Pinchot S, Chen H, Sippel R. Incisions and exposure of the neck for thyroidectomy and parathyroidectomy. Operat Tech Gen Surg 2008;10:63–76.
2. Gagner M. Endoscopic subtotal parathyroidectomy in patients with primary hyperparathyroidism. Br J Surg 1996;83:875.
3. Naitoh T, Gagner M, Garcia-Ruiz A, et al. Endoscopic endocrine surgery in the neck. An initial report of endoscopic subtotal parathyroidectomy. Surg Endosc 1998;12:202–5.
4. Miccoli P, Berti P, Conte M, et al. Minimally invasive surgery for thyroid small nodules: preliminary report. J Endocrinol Invest 1999;22:849–51.
5. Bellantone R, Lombardi CP, Raffaelli M, et al. Minimally invasive, totally gasless video-assisted thyroid lobectomy. Am J Surg 1999;177:342–3.
6. Terris DJ, Seybt MW, Elchoufi M, et al. Cosmetic thyroid surgery: defining the essential principles. Laryngoscope 2007;117:1168–72.

7. Terris DJ, Chin E. Clinical implementation of endoscopic thyroidectomy in selected patients. Laryngoscope 2006;116:1745–8.
8. McCurdy J. Considerations in Asian cosmetic surgery. Facial Plast Surg Clin North Am 2007;15:387–97.
9. Duh Q. Robot-assisted endoscopic thyroidectomy: has the time come to abandon neck incisions? Ann Surg 2011;253(6):1067–8.
10. Ohgami M, Ishii S, Arisawa Y, et al. Scarless endoscopic thyroidectomy: breast approach for better cosmesis. Surg Laparosc Endosc Percutan Tech 2000;10:1–4.
11. Ikeda Y, Takami H, Niimi M, et al. Endoscopic thyroidectomy by the axillary approach. Surg Endosc 2001;15:1362–4.
12. Hüscher CS, Chiodinin S, Napolitano C, et al. Endoscopic right thyroid lobectomy. Surg Endosc 1997;11:877.
13. Gottlieb A, Sprung J, Zheng XM, et al. Massive subcutaneous emphysema and severe hypercarbia in a patient during endoscopic transcervical parathyroidectomy using carbon dioxide insufflation. Anesth Analg 1997;84:1154–6.
14. Miccoli P, Berti P, Raffaelli M, et al. Minimally invasive video-assisted thyroidectomy. Am J Surg 2001;181:567–70.
15. Shimizu K, Akira S, Tanaka S. Video-assisted neck surgery: endoscopic resection of benign thyroid tumor aiming at scarless surgery on the neck. J Surg Oncol 1998;69:178–80.
16. Kataoka H, Kitano H, Takeuchi E, et al. Total video endoscopic thyroidectomy via the anterior chest approach using the cervical region-lifting method. Biomed Pharmacother 2002;56:68s–71s.
17. Youben F, Bo W, Chunlin Z, et al. Trans-areola single-site endoscopic thyroidectomy: pilot study of 35 cases. Surg Endosc 2012;26:939–47.
18. Kang SW, Lee SC, Lee SH, et al. Robotic thyroid surgery using a gasless, transaxillary approach and the da Vinci S system: the operative outcomes of 338 consecutive patients. Surgery 2009;146:1048–55.
19. Rosato L, Avenia N, Bernante P, et al. Complications of thyroid surgery: analysis of a multicentric study on 14,934 patients operated on in Italy over 5 years. World J Surg 2004;28:271–6.
20. Gupta PK, Smith RB, Gupta H, et al. Outcomes after thyroidectomy and parathyroidectomy. Head Neck 2012;34:477–84.
21. Miccoli P, Berti P, Materazzi G, et al. Minimally invasive video-assisted thyroidectomy: five years of experience. J Am Coll Surg 2004;199:243–8.
22. Terris DJ, Angelos P, Steward DL, et al. Minimally invasive video-assisted thyroidectomy. A multi-institutional North American experience. Arch Otolaryngol Head Neck Surg 2008;134:81–4.
23. Park CS, Chung WY, Chang HS. Minimally invasive open thyroidectomy. Surg Today 2001;31:665–9.
24. Tan CT, Cheah WK, Delbridge L. "Scarless" (in the neck) endoscopic thyroidectomy (SET): an evidence-based review of published techniques. World J Surg 2008;32:1349–57.
25. Kang SW, Jeong JJ, Yun JS, et al. Robot-assisted endoscopic surgery for thyroid cancer: experience with the first 100 patients. Surg Endosc 2009;23:2399–406.
26. Jackson NR, Yao L, Tufano RP, et al. Safety of robotic thyroidectomy approaches: meta-analysis and systematic review. Head Neck 2013;36:137–43. http://dx.doi.org/10.1002/hed.23223.
27. Lee J, Yun JH, Nam KH, et al. The learning curve for robotic thyroidectomy: a multicenter study. Ann Surg Oncol 2011;18:226–32.

28. Landry C, Grubbs E, Warneke C, et al. Robot-assisted transaxillary thyroid surgery in the United States: is it comparable to open thyroid lobectomy? Ann Surg Oncol 2012;19:1269–74.
29. Cabot JC, Lee CR, Brunaud L, et al. Robotic and endoscopic transaxillary thyroidectomies may be cost prohibitive when compared to standard cervical thyroidectomy: a cost analysis. Surgery 2012;152:1016–24.
30. Perrier N. Why i have abandoned robot-assisted transaxillary thyroid surgery. Surgery 2012;152:1025–6.
31. Minuto MN, Berti P, Miccoli M, et al. Minimally invasive video-assisted thyroidectomy: an analysis of results and a revision of indications. Surg Endosc 2012;26: 818–22.
32. Neidich MJ, Steward DL. Safety and feasibility of elective minimally invasive video-assisted central neck dissection for thyroid carcinoma. Head Neck 2012;34:354–8.
33. Miccoli P, Bellantone R, Mourad M, et al. Minimally invasive video-assisted thyroidectomy: multiinstitutional experience. World J Surg 2002;26:972–5.
34. Miccoli P, Elisei R, Materazzi G, et al. Minimally invasive video-assisted thyroidectomy for papillary carcinoma: a prospective study of its completeness. Surgery 2002;132:1070–4.
35. Terris DJ, Seybt MW. Modifications of Miccoli minimally invasive thyroidectomy for the low-volume surgeon. Am J Otolaryngol 2011;32:392–7.
36. Ferzli GS, Sayad P, Abdo Z, et al. Minimally invasive, nonendoscopic thyroid surgery. J Am Coll Surg 2001;192:665–8.
37. Cavicchi O, Piccin O, Rinaldi A, et al. Minimally invasive nonendoscopic thyroidectomy. Otolaryngol Head Neck Surg 2006;135:744–7.
38. Hur SM, Kim SH, Lee SK, et al. New endoscopic thyroidectomy with the bilateral areolar approach: a comparison with the bilateral axillo-breast approach. Surg Laparosc Endosc Percutan Tech 2011;21:e219–24.
39. Youben F, Bomin G, Bo W, et al. Trans-areola single-incision endoscopic thyroidectomy. Surg Laparosc Endosc Percutan Tech 2011;21:e192–6.
40. Shimazu K, Shiba E, Tamaki Y, et al. Endoscopic thyroid surgery through the axillo-bilateral-breast approach. Surg Laparosc Endosc Percutan Tech 2003; 13:196–201.
41. Yeung GH. Endoscopic thyroid surgery today: a diversity of surgical strategies. Thyroid 2002;12:703–6.
42. Ogden J, Lindridge L. The impact of breast scarring on perceptions of attractiveness. An experimental study. J Health Psychol 2008;13:303–10.
43. Ikeda Y, Takami H, Sasaki Y, et al. Clinical benefits in endoscopic thyroidectomy by the axillary approach. J Am Coll Surg 2003;196:189–95.
44. Yoon JH, Park CH, Chung WO. Gasless endoscopic thyroidectomy via an axillary approach: experience of 30 Cases. Surg Laparosc Endosc Percutan Tech 2006;16:226–31.
45. Kang SW, Jeong JJ, Nam KH, et al. Robot-assisted endoscopic thyroidectomy for thyroid malignancies using a gasless transaxillary approach. J Am Coll Surg 2009;209:e1–7.
46. Choe JH, Kim SW, Chung KW, et al. Endoscopic thyroidectomy using a new bilateral axillo-breast approach. World J Surg 2007;31:601–6.
47. Bärlehner E, Benhidjeb T. Cervical scarless endoscopic thyroidectomy: axillo-bilateral-breast approach (ABBA). Surg Endosc 2008;22:154–7.
48. Lobe T, Wright SK, Irish MS. Novel uses of surgical robotics in head and neck surgery. J Laparoendosc Adv Surg Tech A 2005;15:647–52.

49. Lee KE, Rao J, Youn YK. Endoscopic thyroidectomy with the da Vinci robot system using the bilateral axillary breast approach (BABA) technique. Our initial experience. Surg Laparosc Endosc Percutan Tech 2009;19:e71–5.
50. Ryu HR, Kang SW, Lee SH, et al. Feasibility and safety of a new robotic thyroidectomy through a gasless, transaxillary single-incision approach. J Am Coll Surg 2010;211:e13–9.
51. Terris DJ, Singer MC, Seybt MW. Robot facelift thyroidectomy: II. Clinical feasibility and safety. Laryngoscope 2011;121:1636–41.
52. Kang SW, Park JH, Jeong JS, et al. Prospects of robotic thyroidectomy using a gasless, transaxillary approach for the management of thyroid carcinoma. Surg Laparosc Endosc Percutan Tech 2011;21:223–9.
53. Tae KT, Ji YB, Cho SH, et al. Early surgical outcomes of robotic thyroidectomy by a gasless unilateral axillo-breast or axillary approach for papillary thyroid carcinoma: 2 years' experience. Head Neck 2012;34:617–25.
54. Dionigi G. Robotic thyroidectomy: seoul is not varese. Otolaryngol Head Neck Surg 2013;148:178.
55. Kuppersmith R, Holsinger F. Robotic thyroid surgery: an initial experience with North American patients. Laryngoscope 2011;121:521–6.
56. Kandil E, Noureldine S, Yao L, et al. Robotic transaxillary thyroidectomy: an examination of the first one hundred cases. J Am Coll Surg 2012;214:558–66.
57. Inabnet WB. Robotic thyroidectomy: must we drive a luxury sedan to arrive at our destination safely? Thyroid 2012;22:988–90.
58. Terris DJ, Singer MC. Qualitative and quantitative differences between 2 robotic thyroidectomy techniques. Otolaryngol Head Neck Surg 2012;147:20–5.
59. Terris D, Singer MC, Seybt MW. Robotic facelift thyroidectomy: patient selection and technical considerations. Surg Laparosc Endosc Percutan Tech 2011;21(4):237–42.
60. Terris DJ, Singer MC. Robotic facelift thyroidectomy: facilitating remote access surgery. Head Neck 2012;34:746–7.

Management of the Neck in Thyroid Cancer

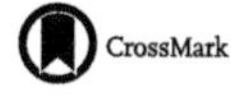

David W. Schoppy, MD, PhD, F. Christopher Holsinger, MD*

KEYWORDS

• Thyroid cancer • Neck dissection • Paratracheal

KEY POINTS

- Surgery should be tailored to achieve the oncologic goals of disease eradication while preserving voice, airway, swallowing, and parathyroid function.
- Although controversial, prophylactic central compartment (level VI) neck dissection for papillary thyroid carcinoma should be considered in certain circumstances (tumors > 4 cm or those with extrathyroidal extension).
- When indicated, functional or modified radical neck dissection for differentiated thyroid cancer generally includes lymphadenectomy of levels IIa, III, IV, and Vb of the neck.
- Empiric oral supplementation with elemental calcium and vitamin D is generally warranted after paratracheal and mediastinal lymph node dissection.

INTRODUCTION

For regional control of differentiated thyroid cancer (DTC), the goal of lymphadenectomy is the complete surgical resection of all grossly evident metastatic disease and the selective removal of regional lymph node groups at highest risk for microscopic disease. Moreover, surgery should be tailored to achieve the oncologic goals of disease eradication while preserving voice, airway, swallowing, and parathyroid function. Therefore, management of the neck or cervical lymphadenectomy is the preferred treatment to obtain regional control in patients with cervical lymph node metastasis detected on initial staging. Likewise, an aggressive surgical approach is warranted for recurrent regional metastasis, because complete resection of disease correlates with improved disease-free survival. This article discusses the central compartment dissection, lateral neck dissection, and dissection of the metastatic retropharyngeal lymphatic node. Preoperative and postoperative care are discussed and a review of the literature is presented to consider new refinements in surgical technique, as well as current controversies and evolving treatment approaches.

Department of Otolaryngology, Stanford University School of Medicine, Stanford Cancer Center, 875 Blake Wilbur Drive, Stanford, CA 94305-5820, USA
* Corresponding author. Division of Head and Neck Surgery, Stanford Cancer Center, 875 Blake Wilbur Drive, CC-2227, Stanford, CA 94304.
E-mail address: holsinger@stanford.edu

Otolaryngol Clin N Am 47 (2014) 545–556
http://dx.doi.org/10.1016/j.otc.2014.04.004 oto.theclinics.com
0030-6665/14/$ – see front matter

LYMPHADENECTOMY FOR THYROID CANCER

Approach to the management of cervical lymph nodes in thyroid cancer is guided by many factors, including the preoperative detection of metastasis.[1,2] Ultrasonography of the central and lateral neck is recommended by the American Thyroid Association (ATA) and current National Comprehensive Cancer Network guidelines during the preoperative evaluation of most thyroid malignancies.[1,3] Papillary carcinoma, the most common histologic subtype of thyroid cancer, is often metastatic to regional lymph nodes on pathologic review,[4,5] and ultrasonography can suggest lymph node involvement in approximately one-third of patients.[6,7] Although ultrasonography is more sensitive than physical examination, a substantial number of patients have microscopic disease found on pathology following neck dissection for clinically negative necks, especially in the central compartment.[8,9] However, ultrasonography may be sufficient for the detection of clinically relevant disease in papillary thyroid carcinomas,[6] and ultrasonography may be especially useful in evaluation of lymph nodes in the lateral neck.[9,10] Preoperative ultrasonography can significantly affect the extent of surgery planned for papillary carcinoma, as well as other types of thyroid malignancies.[11] The preoperative detection of lymph node involvement by either clinical examination or imaging can significantly clarify the goal of neck management and make clear the distinction between a prophylactic and therapeutic neck dissection. In review of current guidelines and existing literature, a therapeutic dissection of clinically apparent node compartments is generally recommended in the surgical management of most thyroid cancers.[1,3,12]

Central Lymph Node Compartment

The central lymph node compartment (level VI) is frequently involved,[13,14] and is bounded laterally by the carotid arteries, the hyoid bone superiorly, and the sternal notch (or the innominate artery if level VII is included) inferiorly (**Fig. 1**).[15] Lymph nodes within this compartment most commonly involved by metastatic thyroid carcinoma include the prelaryngeal (Delphian), pretracheal, and paratracheal nodes.[15] An adequate unilateral central neck dissection, as defined by the ATA, should include the prelaryngeal, pretracheal, and the ipsilateral paratracheal nodal group.[15] If performed with therapeutic intent, it is recommended that the dissection be extended to include bilateral paratracheal nodal groups.[1,16] Other nodes within the central compartment that are less commonly involved include the retropharyngeal, retroesophageal, and paralaryngopharyngeal groups.[15]

Lateral Node Involvement

Although metastatic thyroid carcinoma most frequently involves the central compartment, recent data have shown a high incidence of lateral nodal involvement, with pathologic metastasis in more than half of patients with papillary thyroid cancer[17] and a similarly high number of patients with medullary carcinoma.[13] Level III (ranging from the hyoid bone superiorly to the cricoid cartilage inferiorly and bounded by the sternohyoid medially and posterior border of the sternocleidomastoid laterally) is the most commonly involved lateral cervical group, but meta-analysis data have shown a high prevalence of multilevel disease, with levels II, III, IV, and V having metastatic involvement in 53%, 71%, 66%, and 25% of therapeutic neck dissections respectively for DTCs (see **Fig. 1**).[18] The ATA has further reviewed the lateral neck dissection and recommends a therapeutic dissection of levels IIa, III, IV, and Vb when suspicious nodes are identified before surgery.[19] The morbidity associated with further dissection of level V to include the superior portion of level Va (above the spinal accessory nerve)

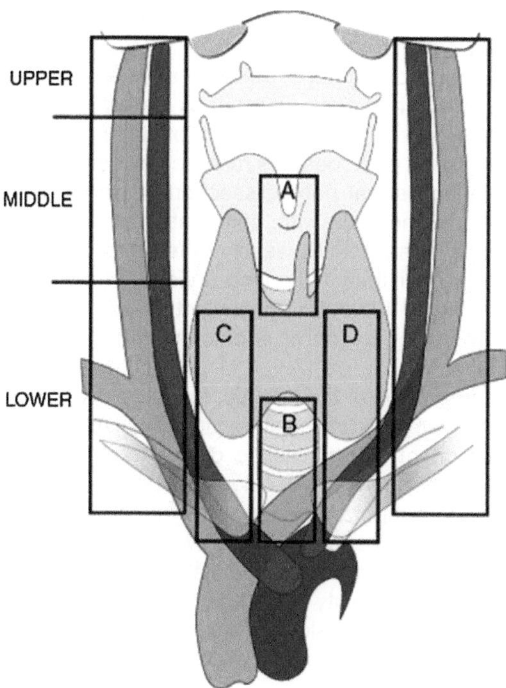

Fig. 1. The 4 major node-bearing regions within the central neck: prelaryngeal (Delphian) (A), pretracheal (B), and bilateral paratracheal (C and D). (*From* Tufano RP, Potenza A, Randolph GW. Central neck dissection. In: Randolph GW, editor. Surgery of the thyroid and parathyroid glands. Philadelphia: Elsevier; 2012; with permission.)

may be spared in the absence of clinically evident disease, because data show that this level is rarely involved.[20,21]

Prophylactic Neck Dissection

Distinct from a therapeutic neck dissection, which most literature suggests is beneficial and generally recommended, is a prophylactic neck dissection, for which the indications are less clear. Existing data are heterogeneous in the demonstrated benefits and any associated morbidity of prophylactic central compartment neck dissection, especially in patients with papillary thyroid carcinoma.[22]

In papillary carcinoma, current guidelines recommend considering a prophylactic central neck dissection if other factors in patient presentation prompt a total thyroidectomy.[3] This position generally agrees with published recommendations from the ATA, which broadly suggest considering a prophylactic central neck dissection, especially in patients with advanced primary tumors larger than 4 cm.[1] Again, papillary thyroid cancer is frequently metastatic to regional lymph nodes.[4,5] In addition, the presence of lymph node metastasis may not be readily apparent on preoperative evaluation.[8,9,23] However, the significance of this nodal involvement is less obvious. Several studies have shown that the pathologic identification of lymph node metastasis in papillary thyroid cancer can help predict disease-free and disease-specific survival and, thus, potentially help guide postoperative management.[24–28] Although a prophylactic central lymph node dissection can offer information regarding prognosis, it is unclear whether it can be therapeutic. A review of literature documenting locoregional recurrence rates in clinically N0 patients with papillary thyroid carcinoma who underwent either total thyroidectomy (TT) alone or TT with concurrent prophylactic central neck dissections detailed a significant decrease (4.7% vs 8.6%) in recurrence rates when neck dissections were performed.[29] However, this effect may be contributed to by an advancement of staging with pathologic information and an increased use of postoperative radioactive iodine (RAI).[29] In addition, the benefit of a prophylactic central neck dissection in papillary thyroid cancer has not been uniformly documented, with some studies showing only a marginal decrease in recurrence rates.[30,31] However, other work comparing patients with papillary carcinomas greater than 1 cm who uniformly received postoperative RAI following either TT alone or TT and a prophylactic neck dissection showed lower retreatment rates (either reoperation or additional RAI) in patients who underwent a neck dissection.[32]

Any benefit, either prognostic or therapeutic, to a prophylactic central neck dissection may be partly tempered by associated morbidity. Although some series have shown that the inclusion of a prophylactic central compartment neck dissection only increases the risk of temporary hypocalcemia,[29] other studies have documented an additional increase in temporary recurrent laryngeal nerve paralysis.[31,33] These complications may be more closely associated with concurrent thyroidectomy than with the neck dissection.[34] Regardless, the risks associated with the procedure, viewed in the context of uncertainty with regard to the improvement in outcomes, have led to the suggestion to consider a prophylactic central compartment neck dissection in papillary thyroid carcinomas that are either large tumors (>4 cm) or those with extrathyroidal extension.[1,33]

Subtypes of Papillary Thyroid Carcinoma

There is much interest in further refining the approach to papillary thyroid carcinoma, which may eventually be dictated by molecular analysis of the primary tumor.[33,35] At present, histologic analysis can offer some guidance in management. The different subtypes of papillary thyroid carcinoma are increasingly being recognized as distinct entities with differing biological behavior.

Follicular-variant papillary thyroid carcinoma (FV-PTC) is one of the most common variants of papillary carcinoma.[36,37] It has the nuclear features of papillary carcinoma, but grows in a follicular architecture and has a high frequency of *RAS* point mutations, similar to other follicular carcinomas.[36,37] Most FV-PTCs (excluding infiltrative subtypes) have a lower incidence of lymph node metastasis at presentation than classic papillary thyroid carcinomas.[38–41] Recent literature suggests that a prophylactic central compartment neck dissection may be avoided in FV-PTCs.[38,40] However, most FV-PTCs are diagnosed as such after surgery and other factors distinct from the histologic subtype often guide the decision to perform a prophylactic neck dissection. In select patients who undergo a thyroid lobectomy for papillary thyroid cancer, the diagnosis of FV-PTC may obviate further surgery, including a central neck dissection.[38,42]

In contrast with papillary thyroid carcinoma, follicular thyroid cancer is less frequently metastatic to regional lymph nodes and, as such, a prophylactic central compartment neck dissection is rarely performed. Furthermore, because follicular carcinoma cannot be reliably diagnosed with fine-needle aspiration before surgery, the role of central neck dissection in this disease may be limited. For patients with tumors classified before surgery as follicular neoplasm and found to have cervical metastasis, the surgeon should consider the possibility of FV-PTC rather than the diagnosis of follicular carcinoma. Routine prophylactic central neck dissections for follicular carcinomas are therefore not recommended.[3]

Hürthle cell carcinoma, an aggressive variant of follicular carcinoma, is often locally recurrent following primary resection with definitive intent.[43] Similar to papillary thyroid carcinoma, current literature and recommendations support a therapeutic central and/or lateral compartment neck dissection for clinically involved nodes in Hürthle cell carcinoma and suggest considering a prophylactic central compartment neck dissection if a TT is prompted by other factors.[3,44]

Medullary thyroid cancer is often metastatic to regional lymph nodes at presentation.[45] In contrast with papillary thyroid cancer, in which the role of a prophylactic central neck dissection in the context of a clinically negative neck is less clear, routine central compartment neck dissection is recommended for patients with sporadic medullary thyroid cancer greater than 1 cm or patients with bilateral thyroid disease.[3,12] Lateral neck dissection may be reserved for patients with clinically evident disease on preoperative examination or imaging.[46] However, the presence of lateral cervical disease may not always be obvious before or even during surgery.[13,47] In addition, there is a high rate of lateral cervical compartment microscopic disease in patients with involvement of the central compartment. Although patients with no pathologic involvement of the central neck have a low rate of lateral neck metastasis (10%), patients with even limited central involvement (1–3 positive nodes) have a high rate of lateral compartment disease.[48] Thus, some clinicians have advocated for prophylactic lateral neck dissection when medullary carcinoma has spread to the central lymph node compartment.[12,47]

SURGICAL TECHNIQUE

Central Compartment Dissection (Levels VI and VII)

Dissection of the central compartment includes lymphadenectomy of the pretracheal, paratracheal, and anterior mediastinal lymphoadipose tissues, all of which represent a potential first echelon of nodal drainage from the thyroid gland.[15] Central compartment dissection is performed to remove clinically involved nodes or those at risk for metastatic disease based on features of the primary tumor.

For patients with papillary thyroid cancer, routine prophylactic central compartment dissection is not recommended. However, the thyroid surgeon should inspect and assess at-risk nodal echelons during TT and biopsy with frozen section any suspicious central compartment node to guide further surgical intervention. For patients with primary tumors greater than 4 cm, or with evidence of local invasion, an elective central compartment dissection may be indicated.[1]

Surgical technique

Central compartment dissection should encompass paratracheal, precricoid, and parathyroidal nodes located along the recurrent laryngeal nerves (level VI), as well as superior mediastinal nodes (level VII) (**Fig. 2**).[49] The craniocaudal extent of a central compartment dissection begins at the innominate artery below and ends at the hyoid bone above.[15] The lateral extent of the central compartment dissection is the medial border of the carotid sheath. There are 3 critical but related objectives for this surgery.

1. Once an indication for central compartment dissection has been confirmed, the surgeon should be as comprehensive as possible in removing nodes
2. Preserve the anatomic integrity
3. Minimize trauma to both the recurrent laryngeal nerves and vascularized parathyroid
    - Central compartment dissection is performed after TT and begins by opening the carotid sheath from the hyoid bone to the proximal common carotid artery.

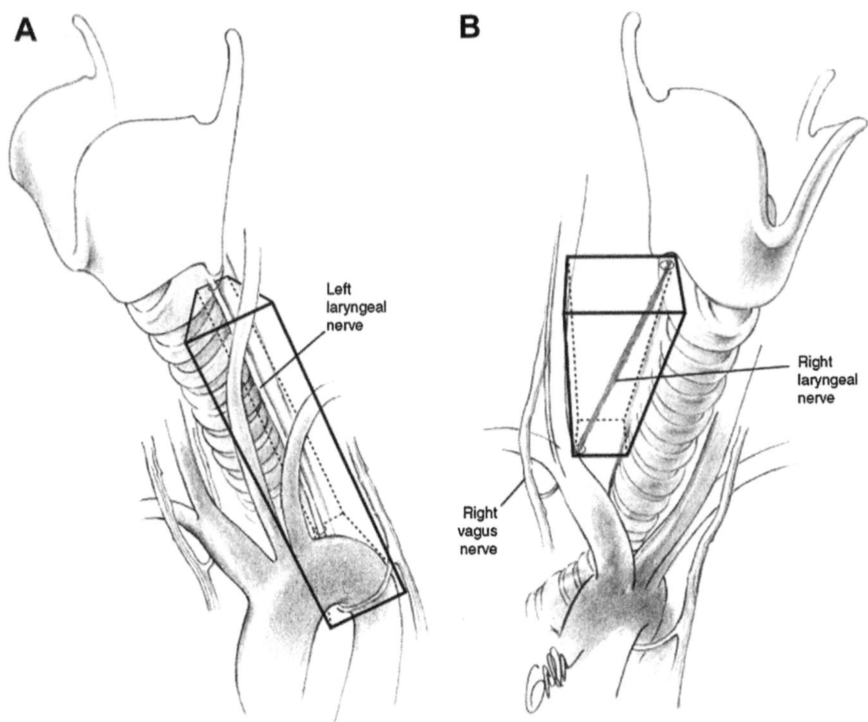

Fig. 2. Varying anatomy of the left versus right paratracheal regions. The nodal compartment on the left (*A*) has greater depth because the nerve enters more ventrally underneath the bifurcating innominate artery, which lies ventral to the trachea. The right nerve then extends medially and ascends to its laryngeal entry point at the right lateral inferior edge of the cricoid cartilage. The right paratracheal region therefore can be divided into 2 triangles: an upper lateral triangle and a lower medial triangle. The nerve divides the compartment into anterior and posterior compartments, and nodes may be deep to the right recurrent laryngeal nerve because of this increased depth of the right paratracheal region compared with the left. This increased depth may require a 360° dissection of the recurrent laryngeal nerve during right paratracheal dissection. The left paratracheal region (*B*) is more flat and two-dimensional because of the tracheoesophageal groove location typical of the left recurrent laryngeal nerve as it traverses this region. (*From* Tufano RP, Potenza A, Randolph GW. Central neck dissection. In: Randolph GW, editor. Surgery of the thyroid and parathyroid glands. Philadelphia: Elsevier; 2012; with permission.)

- In the *right neck*, the dissection is performed down to the origin of the right common carotid artery and its emergence from the brachiocephalic (or innominate) artery.
- The innominate artery is followed until the trachea is encountered.
- The right recurrent laryngeal nerve is identified as it emerges underneath the innominate artery then ascends superiorly from lateral to medial.
- In the *left neck*, because the left common carotid artery arises directly from the aortic arch, this great vessel provides a less reliable guide compared with the right. As a result, the common carotid artery is traced until the trachea is identified, usually at the level of the left brachiocephalic vein.
- The left recurrent laryngeal nerve takes a more medial course, ascending deep to the aortic arch and proximal common carotid artery.

- Upper mediastinal lymphoadipose tissue is then mobilized, because thyrothymic and the inferior thyroid veins must be individually clamped and ligated.
- This specimen is then swept superiorly to begin mobilizing the specimen.

Surgical Notes: For optimal postoperative parathyroid function, the surgeon must maintain and protect the inferior thyroid artery. If the resection of the tumor permits, preserving the superior parathyroid glands usually results in the best chance for long-term normal parathyroid function. The superior parathyroid has a more consistent location in its association with the superior, posteromedial aspect of the thyroid gland. The more variable location of the inferior parathyroid gland may be associated with greater difficulty in preserving this gland with a robust blood supply intact. Furthermore, nodes in the tracheoesophageal groove often place the inferior parathyroid at risk. If the vascularity of either parathyroid gland is compromised, autotransplantation into the ipsilateral sternocleidomastoid muscle should be performed.

- With the ipsilateral nerve circumferentially dissected and with at least one vascularized parathyroid preserved, the remaining lymphadipose tissue is removed.
- Small-caliber vessels are managed with bipolar electrocautery, whereas larger vessels are suture ligated. The use of clips in this area is not recommended, because this practice confounds future computed tomography imaging of the paratracheal bed as well as future surgical intervention.

Modified Radical Neck Dissection (Levels II, III, IV, and V)

Functional or modified radical neck dissection for DTC includes lymphadenectomy of levels II, III, IV, and V of the neck, with preservation of the sternocleidomastoid muscle, internal jugular vein, and spinal accessory nerve. Direct invasion or true nodal fixation is uncommon for metastases of DTC and fascial planes are generally well preserved. Therefore, sacrifice of neurovascular structures during neck dissection is not often necessary. As a result, a comprehensive or modified radical neck dissection should be performed with the expectation of normal postoperative shoulder, swallowing, and sensory function. Superselective neck dissections or nodal berry-picking procedures are associated with unacceptably high levels of disease recurrence in the neck and should not be performed.

Surgical technique

Neck dissection can be performed by extending laterally the transverse Kocher incision and then curving the incision superiorly, ideally behind the line of the posterior border of the sternocleidomastoid muscle. The length of this vertical limb varies, based on the length of the patient's neck, but should always facilitate good exposure of level IIa and IIb. Level IIb is not dissected but access to the lymphatics tracking along the superior thyroid lymphovascular tree is important.

- After subplatysmal flaps are elevated, the superficial layer of the deep cervical fascia is then incised to define the borders of the dissection.
- The fascia is incised inferior to the submandibular gland to identify the digastric tendon and the posterior belly of the digastric muscle.
- The fascial incision is then carried to just below the submandibular gland above to inferiorly along the posterior border of the sternocleidomastoid muscle to the clavicle.
- Fibrofatty tissue lateral to the sternohyoid and sternothyroid muscles is especially dissected here, because metastasis from DTC can be concealed within the folds of these muscles, especially because these muscles insert below onto the clavicle.

- Then, lateral retraction of the sternocleidomastoid provides wide access to levels II to IV.
- High in the neck, the spinal accessory nerve is preserved, with careful dissection of lymphoadipose tissue overlying the nerve.
- For patients with known level IIa metastasis, level IIb dissection has been advocated.[50] A careful dissection then mobilizes the lymphatic tissues associated with levels II to IV from the jugular vein and carotid artery.

Surgical Notes: Careful attention must be paid to the route of common metastatic spread: along the superior thyroid artery and the transverse cervical artery. Small nodes can be missed if the surgeon is rushed or not systematic in the dissection of this crucial area.

- Dissection in the posterior triangle is most often limited to level Vb along the transverse cervical lymphovascular system.
- As the sternocleidomastoid muscle (SCM) is retracted medially, the spinal accessory nerve is identified as it emerges from the posterior border of the SCM at the junction of the superior third and lower two-thirds of the muscle, usually within 1 cm of the Erb point.
- The nerve is then dissected circumferentially to its entrance in the trapezius muscle, which is usually 1 to 2 cm above the clavicle.
- Before closure, the wound should be thoroughly irrigated with saline and complete hemostasis achieved.

Surgical Notes: A Valsalva maneuver can elicit lymphatic or venous sources of oozing. Powdered microfibrillar collagen (Avitene) may help to control bleeding from raw surfaces, especially in the anterior mediastinum.

- Flat, fully fluted, 7-mm closed suction drains are placed in the central and lateral neck compartments.
- Absorbable gelatin (Gelfoam) may be used to cover the recurrent or spinal accessory nerves and protect the direct contact of suctioning drains.
- After neck dissection and TT, serum levels of calcium, phosphorous, albumin, magnesium, and intact parathyroid hormone (iPTH) are assessed immediately after surgery and then subsequently until serum calcium homeostasis is achieved.
- Surgical drain(s) in the neck are removed when daily output decreases to less than 30 mL over a 24-hour period.

POSTOPERATIVE CARE AND MANAGEMENT

Hypoparathyroidism and Hypocalcemia

The extent of vascularized parathyroid tissue preserved at operation predicts the probability of postoperative hypocalcemia. Moreover, serum iPTH levels in the early postoperative period strongly predict glandular function. Although levels of iPTH in the normal range can be reassuring, those in a low but detectable range predict a higher probability of transient or permanent hypocalcemia. Moreover, undetectable iPTH levels are strongly correlated with hypocalcemia requiring intravenous infusion of calcium gluconate in the postoperative period. Empiric oral supplementation with elemental calcium and vitamin D is generally warranted after paratracheal and mediastinal lymph node dissection. Intravenous calcium gluconate is reserved for patients with symptomatic hypocalcemia manifest by perioral numbness or tingling in the fingers or toes. An infusion can be delivered by adding 10 ampoules of calcium gluconate to a 500-mL of normal saline and beginning at 30 mL/h, titrating up as needed to control symptoms.

Recurrent Laryngeal Nerve Injury

Preoperative and postoperative laryngoscopy must be performed by surgeons who operate on the thyroid.[51] Randolph and Kamani[52] showed that the absence of voice disturbance does not guarantee normal nerve function; vocal cord paralysis (identified by laryngoscopy) is more sensitive at identifying recurrent laryngeal nerve defects caused by invasive thyroid malignancy. In the presence of a functional recurrent laryngeal nerve, anatomic preservation of the nerve and its branches is an important component of thyroid surgery.[51] There are several variant extralaryngeal branching patterns that the surgeon must be vigilant for during thyroidectomy and any associated neck dissection.[53] Dissection about the recurrent nerves can result in vocal cord paralysis that is usually transient. Permanent paralysis is rare in the absence of overt nerve injury or transection.[31,33]

Spinal Accessory Nerve Rehabilitation

Even after preservation of the spinal accessory nerve, circumferential dissection can lead to devascularization and subsequent fibrosis. Therefore, early, if not immediate, postoperative rehabilitation is mandatory especially when level II-b is dissected. Close collaboration with physical therapy is essential to track progress and to ensure that the upper two-thirds of the trapezius muscle are being adequately rehabilitated.

Chyle Leak

Metastases from thyroid cancer have a propensity to lie adjacent to the transverse cervical and/or thyrocervical trunk and often inferiorly in level IV, medially. Therefore, injury to the thoracic duct in the left neck or the accessory lymphatic duct in the right can result in a chyle fistula. When dissecting lymphoadipose tissue low in the neck near the proximal internal jugular vein, caudal to the omohyoid muscle, meticulous surgical technique is necessary to avoid this complication. In particular, the area behind the internal jugular vein, over the scalene musculature, can hide small channels from the main trunk of either thoracic lymphatic duct. Here, all fibrofatty lymphatic tissue should be meticulously dissected, clamped, sharply divided, and ligated to avoid injury that might go unrecognized during surgery. If a well-arborized system of the thoracic duct is encountered, intraoperative assessment for the leakage of chyle should be performed. Although a Valsalva maneuver to 40 mm Hg for 1 to 5 seconds can sometimes be helpful, maneuvers to increase intra-abdominal pressure are most effective in identifying an occult leak. If chyle is noted after surgery within a surgical drain, a low-fat medium-chain triglyceride diet should be instituted immediately. A pressure dressing should be applied to the neck. Using these conservative measures, most chyle fistulas resolve spontaneously within a week to 10 days. In rare cases, exploration of the neck is required or videothoracoscopic ligation of the thoracic duct in the chest.

Injury of the Common Carotid Artery

Injury to the carotid artery can occur during dissection of lymph nodes adherent to, or invasive of, the vessel adventitia. However, this complication is rare and is more often encountered in the setting of previously operated neck. Careful preoperative assessment of imaging should alert the surgeon to the potential for such injury: for instance, for nodes found in the retrocarotid and carotid-vertebral notch. In cases such as these it is wise to have atraumatic vascular clamps, such as the Satinsky clamp, in the surgical field.

SUMMARY

Managing the neck effectively and carefully is an essential element in the overall treatment of DTC. With thorough preoperative evaluation, the thyroid surgeon can provide optimal regional lymphadenectomy with minimal morbidity. Ultrasonography plays an increasingly important role in both the preoperative setting, to provide the best operative planning, and for postoperative management and surveillance.

REFERENCES

1. Cooper DS, Doherty GM, Haugen BR, et al. Revised American Thyroid Association management guidelines for patients with thyroid nodules and differentiated thyroid cancer. Thyroid 2009;19:1167–214.
2. McLeod DS, Sawka AM, Cooper DS. Controversies in primary treatment of low-risk papillary thyroid cancer. Lancet 2013;381:1046–57.
3. NCCN. National Comprehensive Cancer Network Clinical Practice Guideline in Oncology, Thyroid Carcinoma, Version 2.2013.NCCN Guidelines 2.2013 (2013).
4. Attie JN, Khafif RA, Steckler RM. Elective neck dissection in papillary carcinoma of the thyroid. Am J Surg 1971;122:464–71.
5. Noguchi S, Noguchi A, Murakami N. Papillary carcinoma of the thyroid. I. Developing pattern of metastasis. Cancer 1970;26:1053–60.
6. Moreno MA, Edeiken-Monroe BS, Siegel ER, et al. In papillary thyroid cancer, preoperative central neck ultrasound detects only macroscopic surgical disease, but negative findings predict excellent long-term regional control and survival. Thyroid 2012;22:347–55.
7. Roh JL, Kim JM, Park CI. Central cervical nodal metastasis from papillary thyroid microcarcinoma: pattern and factors predictive of nodal metastasis. Ann Surg Oncol 2008;15:2482–6.
8. Ahn JE, Lee JH, Yi JS, et al. Diagnostic accuracy of CT and ultrasonography for evaluating metastatic cervical lymph nodes in patients with thyroid cancer. World J Surg 2008;32:1552–8.
9. Hwang HS, Orloff LA. Efficacy of preoperative neck ultrasound in the detection of cervical lymph node metastasis from thyroid cancer. Laryngoscope 2011;121:487–91.
10. Moreno MA, Agarwal G, de Luna R, et al. Preoperative lateral neck ultrasonography as a long-term outcome predictor in papillary thyroid cancer. Arch Otolaryngol Head Neck Surg 2011;137:157–62.
11. O'Connell K, Yen TW, Quiroz F, et al. The utility of routine preoperative cervical ultrasonography in patients undergoing thyroidectomy for differentiated thyroid cancer. Surgery 2013;154:697–701 [discussion: 701–3].
12. Kloos RT, Eng C, Evans DB, et al. Medullary thyroid cancer: management guidelines of the American Thyroid Association. Thyroid 2009;19:565–612.
13. Moley JF, DeBenedetti MK. Patterns of nodal metastases in palpable medullary thyroid carcinoma: recommendations for extent of node dissection. Ann Surg 1999;229:880–7 [discussion: 887–8].
14. Wada N, Duh QY, Sugino K, et al. Lymph node metastasis from 259 papillary thyroid microcarcinomas: frequency, pattern of occurrence and recurrence, and optimal strategy for neck dissection. Ann Surg 2003;237:399–407.
15. Carty SE, Cooper DS, Doherty GM, et al. Consensus statement on the terminology and classification of central neck dissection for thyroid cancer. Thyroid 2009;19:1153–8.

16. Orloff LA, Kuppersmith RB. American Thyroid Association's central neck dissection terminology and classification for thyroid cancer consensus statement. Otolaryngol Head Neck Surg 2010;142:4–5.
17. Mulla MG, Knoefel WT, Gilbert J, et al. Lateral cervical lymph node metastases in papillary thyroid cancer: a systematic review of imaging-guided and prophylactic removal of the lateral compartment. Clin Endocrinol (Oxf) 2012;77:126–31.
18. Eskander A, Merdad M, Freeman JL, et al. Pattern of spread to the lateral neck in metastatic well-differentiated thyroid cancer: a systematic review and meta-analysis. Thyroid 2013;23:583–92.
19. Stack BC Jr, Ferris RL, Goldenberg D, et al. American Thyroid Association consensus review and statement regarding the anatomy, terminology, and rationale for lateral neck dissection in differentiated thyroid cancer. Thyroid 2012;22:501–8.
20. Roh JL, Kim JM, Park CI. Lateral cervical lymph node metastases from papillary thyroid carcinoma: pattern of nodal metastases and optimal strategy for neck dissection. Ann Surg Oncol 2008;15:1177–82.
21. Khafif A, Medina JE, Robbins KT, et al. Level V in therapeutic neck dissections for papillary thyroid carcinoma. Head Neck 2013;35:605–7.
22. Mazzaferri EL, Doherty GM, Steward DL. The pros and cons of prophylactic central compartment lymph node dissection for papillary thyroid carcinoma. Thyroid 2009;19:683–9.
23. Kim E, Park JS, Son KR, et al. Preoperative diagnosis of cervical metastatic lymph nodes in papillary thyroid carcinoma: comparison of ultrasound, computed tomography, and combined ultrasound with computed tomography. Thyroid 2008;18:411–8.
24. Beasley NJ, Lee J, Eski S, et al. Impact of nodal metastases on prognosis in patients with well-differentiated thyroid cancer. Arch Otolaryngol Head Neck Surg 2002;128:825–8.
25. Leboulleux S, Rubino C, Baudin E, et al. Prognostic factors for persistent or recurrent disease of papillary thyroid carcinoma with neck lymph node metastases and/or tumor extension beyond the thyroid capsule at initial diagnosis. J Clin Endocrinol Metab 2005;90:5723–9.
26. Lundgren CI, Hall P, Dickman PW, et al. Clinically significant prognostic factors for differentiated thyroid carcinoma: a population-based, nested case-control study. Cancer 2006;106:524–31.
27. Podnos YD, Smith D, Wagman LD, et al. The implication of lymph node metastasis on survival in patients with well-differentiated thyroid cancer. Am Surg 2005;71:731–4.
28. Smith VA, Sessions RB, Lentsch EJ. Cervical lymph node metastasis and papillary thyroid carcinoma: does the compartment involved affect survival? Experience from the SEER database. J Surg Oncol 2012;106:357–62.
29. Lang BH, Ng SH, Lau LL, et al. A systematic review and meta-analysis of prophylactic central neck dissection on short-term locoregional recurrence in papillary thyroid carcinoma after total thyroidectomy. Thyroid 2013;23:1087–98.
30. Shan CX, Zhang W, Jiang DZ, et al. Routine central neck dissection in differentiated thyroid carcinoma: a systematic review and meta-analysis. Laryngoscope 2012;122:797–804.
31. Zetoune T, Keutgen X, Buitrago D, et al. Prophylactic central neck dissection and local recurrence in papillary thyroid cancer: a meta-analysis. Ann Surg Oncol 2010;17:3287–93.
32. Hartl DM, Mamelle E, Borget I, et al. Influence of prophylactic neck dissection on rate of retreatment for papillary thyroid carcinoma. World J Surg 2013;37:1951–8.

33. Mehta V, Nathan CA. Prophylactic neck dissection in papillary thyroid cancer: When is it necessary? Laryngoscope 2013;123:2339–40.
34. Cheah WK, Arici C, Ituarte PH, et al. Complications of neck dissection for thyroid cancer. World J Surg 2002;26:1013–6.
35. Joo JY, Park JY, Yoon YH, et al. Prediction of occult central lymph node metastasis in papillary thyroid carcinoma by preoperative BRAF analysis using fine-needle aspiration biopsy: a prospective study. J Clin Endocrinol Metab 2012;97:3996–4003.
36. Asa SL, Mete O. Thyroid neoplasms of follicular cell derivation: a simplified approach. Semin Diagn Pathol 2013;30:178–85.
37. Sebastian SO, Gonzalez JM, Paricio PP, et al. Papillary thyroid carcinoma: prognostic index for survival including the histological variety. Arch Surg 2000;135:272–7.
38. Lin HW, Bhattacharyya N. Clinical behavior of follicular variant of papillary thyroid carcinoma: presentation and survival. Laryngoscope 2010;120:712–6.
39. Passler C, Prager G, Scheuba C, et al. Follicular variant of papillary thyroid carcinoma: a long-term follow-up. Arch Surg 2003;138:1362–6.
40. Salter KD, Andersen PE, Cohen JI, et al. Central nodal metastases in papillary thyroid carcinoma based on tumor histologic type and focality. Arch Otolaryngol Head Neck Surg 2010;136:692–6.
41. Vivero M, Kraft S, Barletta JA. Risk stratification of follicular variant of papillary thyroid carcinoma. Thyroid 2013;23:273–9.
42. Liu J, Singh B, Tallini G, et al. Follicular variant of papillary thyroid carcinoma: a clinicopathologic study of a problematic entity. Cancer 2006;107:1255–64.
43. Stojadinovic A, Ghossein RA, Hoos A, et al. Hurthle cell carcinoma: a critical histopathologic appraisal. J Clin Oncol 2001;19:2616–25.
44. Yutan E, Clark OH. Hurthle cell carcinoma. Curr Treat Options Oncol 2001;2:331–5.
45. Scollo C, Baudin E, Travagli JP, et al. Rationale for central and bilateral lymph node dissection in sporadic and hereditary medullary thyroid cancer. J Clin Endocrinol Metab 2003;88:2070–5.
46. Witt RL. What is the treatment of the lateral neck in clinically localized sporadic medullary thyroid cancer? Laryngoscope 2010;120:1286–7.
47. Moley JF. Medullary thyroid carcinoma: management of lymph node metastases. J Natl Compr Canc Netw 2010;8:549–56.
48. Machens A, Hauptmann S, Dralle H. Prediction of lateral lymph node metastases in medullary thyroid cancer. Br J Surg 2008;95:586–91.
49. Randolph GW. Surgery of the thyroid and parathyroid glands. In: Randolph GW, editor. 2nd edition. Philadelphia: Elsevier Saunders; 2012.
50. Pingpank JF Jr, Sasson AR, Hanlon AL, et al. Tumor above the spinal accessory nerve in papillary thyroid cancer that involves lateral neck nodes: a common occurrence. Arch Otolaryngol Head Neck Surg 2002;128:1275–8.
51. Chandrasekhar SS, Randolph GW, Seidman MD, et al. Clinical practice guideline: improving voice outcomes after thyroid surgery. Otolaryngol Head Neck Surg 2013;148:S1–37.
52. Randolph GW, Kamani D. The importance of preoperative laryngoscopy in patients undergoing thyroidectomy: voice, vocal cord function, and the preoperative detection of invasive thyroid malignancy. Surgery 2006;139:357–62.
53. Cernea CR, Hojaij FC, De Carlucci D Jr, et al. Recurrent laryngeal nerve: a plexus rather than a nerve? Arch Otolaryngol Head Neck Surg 2009;135:1098–102.

Clinical Application of Molecular Testing of Fine-needle Aspiration Specimens in Thyroid Nodules

CrossMark

Linwah Yip, MD[a], Robert L. Ferris, MD, PhD[b,*]

KEYWORDS

• Thyroid cancer • Thyroid nodule • Indeterminate biopsy • Molecular testing

KEY POINTS

- Distinct genetic alterations involving the mitogen-activated protein kinase and phosphatidylinositol 3 kinase pathways characterize thyroid cancer subtypes, and can be detected in preoperative fine-needle aspiration biopsy specimens.
- Identification of these gene mutations and rearrangements can improve the diagnostic utility of preoperative testing, particularly for nodules that are cytologically indeterminate.
- Mutation testing also adds preoperative prognostic information including the identification of thyroid cancers that have a high risk of aggressive histopathologic features, which may further guide the extent of initial thyroidectomy and lymphadenectomy.

INTRODUCTION

Thyroid cancer is the most common endocrine malignancy, its incidence is steadily growing, and it is currently the fifth most common cancer diagnosed in women.[1] Thyroid cancer is typically diagnosed during the evaluation of thyroid nodules, which are highly prevalent in the general population. The incidence of nodule detection has been increasing as the population ages, and as high-resolution diagnostic imaging is increasingly being used.[2] Although most thyroid nodules are benign, the challenge is to accurately and effectively identify malignant nodules. As a standard diagnostic approach, current evidence-based guidelines recommend ultrasonography evaluation with ultrasonography-guided fine-needle aspiration biopsy (FNAB) of thyroid nodules for cytologic examination.[3,4] However in approximately 25% of nodules, the

[a] Endocrine Surgery and Surgical Oncology, Department of Surgery, University of Pittsburgh, 200 Lothrop Street, Pittsburgh, PA 15213, USA; [b] Head and Neck Surgery, Department of Otolaryngology, University of Pittsburgh Cancer Institute, University of Pittsburgh, 200 Lothrop Street, Pittsburgh, PA 15213, USA

* Corresponding author.

E-mail address: ferrrl@upmc.edu

Otolaryngol Clin N Am 47 (2014) 557–571

http://dx.doi.org/10.1016/j.otc.2014.04.003

0030-6665/14/$ – see front matter

cytology is indeterminate, which limits the clinical management.[5] Several molecular testing techniques have been investigated in an attempt to improve diagnostic accuracy. This article focuses on the diagnostic utility of testing for somatic mutations and rearrangements commonly found in thyroid cancer, discusses how preoperative testing can affect operative management, and examines how recently introduced technologies such as next-generation sequencing (NGS) can further expand the diagnostic capability of preoperative FNAB.

Before the routine use of thyroid nodule FNAB, malignancy was found in only 14% of resected thyroid glands.[6] In a recent meta-review, ultrasonography guidance improved diagnostic sensitivity of FNAB to 95%, but the specificity remained low at 47%.[7] When FNAB cytology has adequate cellularity, the results are classified into one of 3 categories: benign, malignant, and indeterminate. FNAB results that are benign or positive for malignancy are often accurate, with false-negative and false-positive rates of 3% to 4% and 1% to 2%, respectively.[8] However, 13% to 40% can be classified as indeterminate, which represents the limitations of cytologic analysis.[3] Indeterminate FNAB results have been further subdivided by the National Cancer Institute in the widely accepted 2007 Bethesda Classification System (**Table 1**) into the following 3 categories: (1) suspicious for malignancy, (2) follicular neoplasm (FN), and (3) follicular lesion of undetermined significance (FLUS)/atypia of undetermined significance (AUS).[9] The suspicious category represents 3% of all FNAB results, and up to 75% prove to be malignant. Morphologic criteria for an FN result predominantly include a hypercellular aspirate of follicular cells indicating follicular proliferation with or without microfollicles, and the differential diagnosis encompasses follicular adenoma (FA), follicular thyroid carcinoma (FTC), or follicular variant of papillary thyroid carcinoma (fvPTC).[9] The malignancy rate is lower (up to 26%), but cytology results indicating FN currently require the patient to undergo at least thyroid lobectomy for definitive diagnosis.[3] The FLUS/AUS category is the most heterogeneous and represents those cytology specimens that are neither benign nor malignant, but may have a degree of cellular and/or architectural atypia that does not meet morphologic criteria for being FN or suspicious.[9] A repeat FNAB may lead to a benign cytology result in up to 40% of nodules[10,11]; however, the malignancy risk is as high as 16% and diagnostic surgery may still be necessary.[8] Thus, many patients undergo surgical resection of benign disease resulting in potentially avoidable morbidity as well as suboptimal use of limited health care resources. Improved diagnostic accuracy of FNAB

Table 1
The National Cancer Institute's suggested fine-needle aspiration (FNA) terminology and the risk of malignancy based on the cytopathologic result

FNA Result	Alternate Accepted Nomenclature	Risk of Malignancy (%)
Benign	—	<1
Atypia of undetermined significance	Atypical lesion of undetermined significance, follicular lesion of undetermined significance, indeterminate follicular lesion, atypical follicular lesion	5–15
Neoplasm	Suspicious for neoplasm, follicular neoplasm	20–30
Suspicious for malignancy	—	50–75
Malignant	—	100
Nondiagnostic	Unsatisfactory	—

cytology evaluation ideally obviates diagnostic surgery and guides the appropriate extent of initial surgery.

MOLECULAR CAUSES OF THYROID MALIGNANCIES

The identification of molecular pathways known to be implicated in thyroid carcinogenesis has significantly expanded options for developing diagnostic adjuncts. The identification of these somatic mutations and rearrangements has helped to further elucidate the specific genetic alterations that occur during the progression from follicular hyperplasia to well-differentiated carcinoma, and much attention has been directed toward elucidating the molecular signature of the 3 most commonly encountered histologic subtypes, which are difficult to differentiate based on FNAB alone: fvPTC, FTC, and FA.[12] Although the diagnosis of histologic variants such as poorly differentiated and anaplastic thyroid cancers is typically straightforward, identification of markers that may herald development of aggressive biological behavior also contributes to improved preoperative risk stratification.

Papillary Thyroid Carcinoma

The mitogen-activated protein kinase (MAPK) pathway alters signaling pathways, induces cell cycle progression, and is typically activated by receptor tyrosine kinases. However, MAPK-mediated tumorigenesis can also be modulated by alternate oncogenic mechanisms such as methylation, chemokine activation, and alterations in components of the tumor microenvironment.[13] Several mutations comprising components of the MAPK pathway have been documented in the development of papillary thyroid carcinoma (PTC) including *RAS* and *BRAF* mutations, and *RET/PTC* rearrangements.[14] Alterations in this oncogenic pathway have been shown in many different malignancies and targeted therapies inhibiting this pathway have been used effectively for a variety of tumor types (eg, Hodgkin lymphoma, glioblastoma multiforme, squamous cell carcinoma, non–small cell lung cancer, and melanoma).

The most common genetic mutation for PTC is an activating point mutation in the *BRAF* gene, occurring in approximately 45% of all PTC.[14] The mutation that leads to substitution of valine for glutamate at residue 600 (*BRAF* V600E) has been implicated in other tumors including melanoma and, less frequently, colorectal adenocarcinoma. Transgenic mice with thyroid-specific *BRAF* V600E expression develop aggressive and radioiodine-resistant PTC.[15,16] The mutation is more commonly seen in the classic version of PTC and the tall-cell variant, but can also be identified in anaplastic carcinoma, poorly differentiated thyroid cancer, and primary thyroid lymphomas. More importantly, FTC and benign lesions do not carry this mutation, thereby making it a specific diagnostic marker for PTC. In a study of more than 4500 cytology samples, all *BRAF* V600E–positive FNAB specimens were histologic malignancies.[17] *BRAF* K601E is the second most common BRAF mutation identified in thyroid cancer and is more likely to be associated with fvPTC.[18]

RAS mutations are found in approximately 10% to 20% of PTC tumors, and are more commonly encountered in fvPTC and FTC.[19] However, *RAS* mutations can be found in the full spectrum of thyroid neoplasms ranging from benign follicular hyperplasia and FA to anaplastic carcinomas.[14] The *RAS* gene encodes for G proteins that are bound to cell membrane receptors and, when stimulated by extracellular signals, result in cellular dysregulation. Activated *RAS* is bound to guanosine triphosphate (GTP), which is tightly mediated by intrinsic *RAS*-regulated GTPase, leading to the inactive GDP-bound *RAS*. Mutations within *RAS* cause constitutive activation either by inactivating the autocatalytic GTPase function (codon 12 or 13) or increasing the binding affinity for GTP (codon 61). The 3 *RAS* gene isoforms (*NRAS*, *KRAS*, and *HRAS*) can activate both the MAPK and phosphatidylinositol 3 kinase (PI3K) pathways.[13] Mutations resulting in *RAS* activation have been shown in 20% to 25% of all human tumors.[13]

RET proto-oncogene point mutations are classically identified in medullary thyroid carcinoma (MTC) and, when genomic, are associated with MEN2 and familial MTC. However, the role of *RET* rearrangements in PTC has been well documented with more than 10 different types of translocations described that are identified in 10% to 20% of PTC.[20,21] The 3′ tyrosine kinase portion of the *RET* gene fuses with the 5′ of a different gene resulting in ligand-independent dimerization and constitutive activation of effector genes in the MAPK and PI3-AKT pathways. The 2 most common fusion proteins are *RET/PTC1* and *RET/PTC3*, which are paracentric versions with the 5′ domain of 2 genes on chromosome 10: *CCDC6* and *NCOA4*, respectively.[20] A higher incidence of *RET/PTC* rearrangements are seen in patients with PTC with a previous history of radiation exposure (50%–80%) or in young patients (40%–70%).[22–24] *RET/PTC1*-positive tumors show either classic papillary architecture or diffuse sclerosing features, whereas *RET/PTC3* is associated with the solid variant. All of the *RET/PTC* tumor subtypes possess a high rate of lymph node metastases.[25] Using highly sensitive detection methods, nonclonal *RET/PTC* rearrangements have also been identified in up to 45% of benign nodules.[26]

TRK rearrangements are gene fusions of the *NTRK1* receptor tyrosine kinase gene on chromosome 1q22, which is one of at least 3 different genes described to date. These rearrangements can also be found in less than 5% of PTC.[12]

FTC and FA

Genetic alterations in the PI3K-AKT pathway are common in FTC and FA.[13,27] Germline mutations in the *PTEN* gene are responsible for Cowden syndrome, which is characterized by benign and malignant follicular thyroid tumors. Increased expression and activation of AKT was reported in FTC and poorly differentiated thyroid cancer, but has also been observed in all subtypes.[28] Somatic point mutations in *PTEN* are identified in ~10% of FTC, but gene methylation resulting in reduced expression levels may be a more frequent mechanism of *PTEN* loss in follicular thyroid lesions.[13] As previously discussed, *RAS* mutations can also activate the PI3K-AKT pathway, and are found in 40% to 50% of FTC and 20% to 40% of FA.[19] Although benign follicular lesions carrying the *RAS* mutations may be precancerous lesions, the identification of *RAS* is nonspecific for histologic malignancy.

A gene rearrangement leading to the fusion of the thyroid-specific paired domain transcription factor *PAX8* and the peroxisome proliferator-activated receptor gene *PPARγ*, which plays an important role in lipid metabolism, was discovered in FTC in 2000.[29] The *PAX8/PPARγ* rearrangement results in overexpression of the fusion protein, but the carcinogenic mechanism of action is unclear. *PAX8* plays an essential role in thyrocyte development, as well as in the gene expression of the sodium-iodide symporter, thyroglobulin, and the thyroid-stimulating hormone receptor.[30] The fusion protein antagonizes the action of *PPARγ* via a dominant-negative inhibition that has been shown to be a causative agent in FTC in vitro and in vivo tumorigenesis.[31] However, the exact carcinogenic consequence of the *PAX8/PPARγ* fusion protein remains theoretic. *PAX8/PPARγ* translocation is found in 30% to 40% of classic FTC, 2% to 10% of FA, and rarely in fvPTC.[32] *PAX8/PPARγ*- positive FA tends to have positive immunohistochemical staining for markers more consistent with FTC, but does not meet histologic criteria for malignancy. Much like *RAS*-positive FAs, *PAX8/PPARγ*-positive FA may represent carcinomas in situ. *PAX8/PPARγ*-positive

FTCs tend to occur in young patients with tumor characteristics that have solid patterns and vascular invasion.[32]

Poorly Differentiated Thyroid Carcinomas

The progression from differentiated thyroid cancer to poorly differentiated or anaplastic thyroid cancer is less well explicated, and could theoretically be caused by either accumulation of multiple genetic alterations resulting in oncogenic amplification, or coexistent MAPK and PI3K-AKT pathway dysregulation that accelerates the genetic alterations that promote tumor growth. Poorly differentiated thyroid carcinomas (PDTC), although uncommon, display more aggressive behavior than well-differentiated thyroid carcinomas, but are less aggressive than the undifferentiated or anaplastic forms. Histology, immunohistochemistry, and molecular genetic tests reinforce the diagnosis of PDTC. Given the aggressiveness of PDTC and the poor survival rates in patients who undergo surgery alone, a multimodality treatment approach is required.

Although rearrangements are rarely identified in PDTC, point mutations found in differentiated thyroid cancer are well-represented. *BRAF* V600E is present in ~15% to 25% of patients with PDTCs but is rarely found in PDTCs arising from FTC. *RAS* gene alterations (commonly point mutations at *HRAS* codon 12 or 61 and *NRAS* at codon 13) are present in 25% to 35% of PDTCs.[12] *RAS*-induced chromosomal instability may predispose to tumor dedifferentiation, perhaps explaining the increased prevalence of mutant *RAS* in anaplastic thyroid carcinomas. However, mutant *RAS* is unlikely to be solely capable of driving tumor dedifferentiation, given its high prevalence (45%) in patients with differentiated thyroid cancer and in those with benign thyroid adenomas.[12] In contrast, Garcia-Rostan and colleagues[33] stated that histologic dedifferentiation is not necessarily driven by *BRAF* or *RAS* mutations individually, but rather represents the cooperation of multiple genetic alterations that likely stimulate dedifferentiation.

Inactivating point mutations of *TP53* are rarely associated with differentiated thyroid cancers; however, they are highly prevalent (25%–30%) in patients with PDTC and ATC.[12,13] Because *p53* is known as the guardian of the genome, unlike *RAS* and *BRAF* gene alterations, which regulate proliferative signals, *p53* mutations possess an important function in triggering tumor dedifferentiation and evolution to PDTC and ATC. Other gene mutations that are associated with tumor dedifferentiation include point mutations in *PIK3CA* (10%–20%), *CTNNB1* encoding beta-catenin (10%–20%), and *AKT1* (5%–10%).[12]

BIOMARKERS USED FOR TUMOR DETECTION AND PROGNOSTICATION

Several prospective and retrospective studies have shown that the diagnostic accuracy of FNAB can be significantly improved using modern molecular detection techniques to identify genetic alterations. In addition, although most patients with differentiated thyroid cancer fare well, biomarkers have also been shown to provide prognostic information that can be used to guide further management.

Molecular Testing of FNAB Specimens

BRAF

Most studies of biomarker detection in FNAB specimens have focused on the *BRAF* V600E mutation. In a 2009 review, Nikiforova and Nikiforov[14] reported on testing for *BRAF* in 2766 samples from 9 prospective fine-needle aspiration (FNA) studies, 7 retrospective FNAB studies, and 2 studies of research FNAB performed on postoperative thyroid specimens (**Table 2**). In this meta-analysis, all 580 *BRAF*-positive clinical FNAB samples studied prospectively and retrospectively were positive for papillary carcinoma, and there was only 1 reported false-positive sample, obtained by research aspiration of the nodule in a surgically removed thyroid gland, resulting in a false-positive rate of 0.2%.[14] *BRAF* V600E mutation can occasionally be detected in false-negative benign FNAB results from histologic malignancies; however, *BRAF* V600E is less common overall than other gene alterations in cytologically indeterminate FNAB specimens.[18,34] Regardless of cytology category, when preoperative *BRAF* V600E is detected in FNAB testing, a diagnosis of thyroid cancer should be suspected. *BRAF* K601E is less frequently detected, but is associated with indeterminate cytology and indolent histology. In a series of 29 indeterminate FNAB specimens with positive *BRAF* testing, 8 (28%) were *BRAF* K601E with histologic malignancies confirmed in all (100%). Only 1 of the 8 malignancies was a solid variant PTC, whereas the remaining 7 were histologic fvPTC.[18]

RAS

RAS mutations are found in both benign and malignant follicular thyroid neoplasms and are the most frequent mutations detected in cytologically indeterminate FNAB results because of the association with FA, FTC, and fvPTC histologies. In a series of 68 *RAS*-positive FNAB specimens, 93% were cytologically indeterminate. The rate of histologic malignancy was 83% and included 46 fvPTC, 4 FTC, 1 MTC, and 1 anaplastic cancer. Most fvPTC was encapsulated, and lymph node metastasis was uncommon.[35] In another study including 97 indeterminate FNAB specimens, *NRAS*-positive results on multivariate analysis also added diagnostic accuracy to preoperative cytology.[36] Although *RAS* positivity is not 100% predictive of malignancy, detection increases the risk to 80% to 85%, which is often high enough to alter initial surgical management to total thyroidectomy for patients who may otherwise require 2-stage thyroidectomy based on indeterminate cytology.[34] Even if histology is benign, there is the potential for malignant transformation associated with a *RAS*-positive FA and surgical resection may be a reasonable treatment option.

RET/PTC

Among differentiated thyroid cancers, the *RET/PTC* rearrangement is typically associated with PTC. In a retrospective analysis comparing patient-matched FNA and post-thyroidectomy specimens, a *RET/PTC* fusion transcript was present in 50% of the FNA samples, all of which were histologically proven PTC in the surgically removed thyroids.[37] No false-positive results were reported in this study. The results confirmed that *RET/PTC* is a highly specific biomarker for the diagnosis of PTC. In addition, the data suggested that molecular investigation was most informative for aspirates that

Table 2
A review of all thyroid FNA studies using the BRAF mutation before 2009. The results of prospective, retrospective, and FNA studies on surgically removed thyroid specimens are shown. BRAF positivity shows an almost universal correlation with a final pathologic result of PTC

Thyroid FNA Studies	Number of Samples	BRAF Positive	Final Diagnosis in BRAF-positive Samples
Prospective studies	1814	159	PTC, 159 (100%)
Retrospective studies	685	291	PTC, 291 (100%)
FNA on thyroid specimens	267	131	PTC, 130 (99.2%) Hyperplasia, 1 (0.8%)
Total	2766	581	PTC, 580 (99.8%)

would otherwise have been nondiagnostic. In 2 of the 6 histologically proven PTCs that had insufficient aspirate for diagnosis by cytologic examination, the correct diagnosis was made by screening for *RET/PTC* on the FNA samples. Of the 15 indeterminate FNAB that were eventually diagnosed as PTC after surgery, 9 were positive for *RET/PTC*. However, if considering *RET/PTC* alone as the diagnostic biomarker, only 50% of the PTC were identified based on the use of molecular diagnostics with *RET/PTC* as the biomarker. In addition, in this series, using both cytologic analysis and *RET/PTC* detection allowed an increased diagnostic yield, from 12 cases definitively diagnosed by cytologic examination alone to 23 cases diagnosed by cytology and molecular marker amplification.[37]

Panel testing

Individual marker testing lacks sufficient specificity and the optimal diagnostic accuracy with DNA-based testing can be achieved with a panel of markers. Testing FNAB specimens for a panel of mutations including *BRAF*, *RAS*, *RET/PTC*, and *PAX8/PPARγ* was first evaluated in 2 independent single-institution series and was shown to be highly associated with thyroid cancer in 146 cytologically indeterminate FNAB specimens with histologic correlation.[38,39] In these studies, 49% of nodules with an identified mutation had one of the non-*BRAF* mutations, and 97% were diagnosed with histologic thyroid cancer. The largest, prospective study done thus far with cytologic, molecular, and histologic correlation included 513 consecutive cytologically indeterminate FNAB specimens.[34] The malignancy rate was 24%. When *BRAF*, *RET/PTC1*, *PTC3*, or PAX8/PPARγ were detected, the risk of malignancy was nearly 100% regardless of cytology category. *RAS* mutations were detected in 73% of the molecular-positive FNAB specimens, and histologic thyroid cancer was diagnosed in 85%. For indeterminate FNAB, the mutation panel had a sensitivity 61%, negative predictive value 89%, specificity of 98%, and positive predictive value (PPV) 89%.[34]

The primary benefit of the panel was to improve the PPV of preoperative testing (**Table 3**). For patients with molecular-positive FNAB results, the overall risk of malignancy was 89% and total thyroidectomy should be considered as the initial surgical procedure. In a series of 471 patients with FNAB results classified as AUS/FLUS or FN, prospective molecular testing using the mutation panel was associated with a 2.5-fold reduction in 2-stage thyroidectomy for histologic clinically significant thyroid cancer.[40] Furthermore, in hypothetical decision-tree modeling, the significant reduction in unnecessary surgeries offset the added costs of molecular testing and resulted in distributed cost savings.[41] Negative mutation panel results may also reduce malignancy risk to allow modifications to current management algorithms for selected patients. For example, mutation-negative AUS/FLUS nodules have a 5.9% risk of malignancy with no malignancies diagnosed in nodules smaller than 1.8 cm[42] and sonographic surveillance may be an option for patients with this subset of small nodules.

Prognostication Using Biomarkers

Although most well-differentiated thyroid carcinomas have indolent behavior and are easily cured by surgical removal, a minority of tumors can be highly aggressive and difficult to treat. The current classifications rely on clinical characteristics (ie, age, extrathyroidal extension, size, and tumor grade) but do not predict the behavior of a neoplasm with any great accuracy. Mutation testing has also shown some promise in this regard, which may also help guide the initial extent of surgical management.

BRAF V600E mutation has been well studied as a prognostic biomarker for PTC. In a review by Xing,[43] *BRAF* mutations correlated with aggressive tumor characteristics

Table 3
Correlation between the results of mutational analysis in FNA samples and outcome in specific groups of indeterminate cytology

	Histology Malignant	Histology Benign	
AUS/FLUS (n = 247)[a]			
	Histology Malignant (n = 35)	Histology Benign (n = 212)	Sensitivity, 63% Specificity, 99%
Mutation Positive (n = 25)	16 RAS (16 fvPTC) 5 BRAF (4 fvPTC) 1 PAX8/PPARg (1 fvPTC)	3 RAS (3 FA)	PPV, 88% NPV, 94% Accuracy, 94%
Mutation Negative (n = 222)	13 (11 fvPTC, 2 PTC)	209 (166 NH, 42 FA)	
FN or Hürthle Cell Neoplasm/Suspicious for FN (n = 214)[b]			
	Histology Malignant (n = 58)	Histology Benign (n = 156)	Sensitivity, 57% Specificity, 97%
Mutation Positive (n = 38)	2 BRAF (1 PTC, 1 fvPTC) 29 RAS (21 fvPTC, 5 PTC, 3 FTC) 2 PAX8/PPARg (2 fvPTC)	5 RAS (5 FA)	PPV, 87% NPV, 86% Accuracy, 86%
Mutation Negative (n = 176)	25 (16 fvPTC, 3 PTC, 6 FTC)	151 (95 HN, 56 FA)	
Suspicious for Malignant Cells (n = 25)[c]			
	Histology Malignant (n = 28)	Histology Benign (n = 24)	Sensitivity, 68% Specificity, 96%
Mutation Positive (n = 20)	10 BRAF (10 PTC) 7 RAS (6fvPTC, 1 FTC) 1 PAX8/PPARg (1 FTC) 1 RET/PTC (1 PTC)	1 RAS (1 FA)	PPV, 95% NPV, 72% Accuracy, 81%
Mutation Negative (n = 32)	9 (7 PTC, 2 fvPTC)	23 (17 HN, 6 FA)	

Abbreviation: HN, hyperplastic nodule.
[a] Molecular testing reduced observed malignant frequency from 16% to 6%.
[b] Molecular testing reduced observed malignant frequency from 27% to 14%.
[c] Molecular testing reduced observed malignant frequency from 54% to 28%.

such as extrathyroidal extension, advanced tumor stage at presentation, and lymph node or distant metastases. The mutation was further shown to be a poor prognostic indicator when positive in FNAB samples. *BRAF* V600E has also been shown to be an independent predictor of tumor recurrence, even in patients with early stage disease. Elisei and colleagues[44] examined 102 patients with PTC over a median of 15 years, and the *BRAF* V600E mutation was an independent risk factor for tumor-related death. More recently, Xing and colleagues[45] examined a multi-institutional and retrospective series of 1840 patients with PTC with median follow-up of 33 months, and observed an association between *BRAF* V600E and increased disease-specific mortality (hazard ratio, 2.66; 95% confidence interval, 1.3–5.4; $P<.001$). However, in multivariate analysis, the effects of *BRAF* did not seem to be independent of extent of disease at presentation including presence of lymph node metastasis, extrathyroidal extension, and distant metastasis. Therefore the utility of *BRAF* V600E testing may be greatest during preoperative planning and in determining the extent of initial surgery. Given the association with lymph node metastasis, lymph node mapping by high-resolution ultrasonography should be performed before initial surgery.

In the absence of clinical or sonographic lymph node involvement, controversy exists as to whether or not a prophylactic central compartment lymph node dissection

(CCND) should be performed.[46] In single-institution small studies, prophylactic CCND reduced postoperative thyroglobulin levels and may decrease locoregional recurrence rates, although no study has yet shown a reduction in disease-specific mortality.[47–50] In addition, a higher rate of postoperative morbidity, including temporary hypocalcemia, has been observed even when the procedure is performed by high-volume surgeons.[49] *BRAF* V600E–positive PTC has a higher risk of central compartment lymph node metastasis and, in multivariate analysis, *BRAF* remains a potent preoperative predictor of nodal disease.[51,52] Thus, *BRAF* V600E may be one way to identify patients who would best benefit from prophylactic CCND.

Several studies have also reported that *BRAF* V600E in papillary thyroid microcarcinomas (PTMC) correlates with higher rates of both extrathyroidal tumor extension and cervical lymph node metastasis.[53,54] Most PTMC are indolent tumors that are incidentally discovered during the removal of presumed large, benign neoplasms, and are almost universally cured by surgical resection. However, a subset of PTMC can behave aggressively, leading to recurrence and mortality. In a molecular-pathologic score derived from a cohort of PTMC and then validated in an independent cohort, *BRAF* V600E along with histopathologic features including fibrosis, superficial location, and intraglandular tumor spread/multifocality could predict PTMC at higher risk for aggressive behavior.[55]

The role of *RAS* mutation as a prognostic biomarker has not been as clearly delineated. As previously mentioned, this tumor is found in both benign and malignant follicular processes, making it difficult to use it for prognosis. However, there is evidence to suggest that an FA that is *RAS* positive is more likely to be a carcinoma precursor or carcinoma in situ. Some studies have suggested a significant correlation between the *RAS* mutation and metastatic potential of FTC that may be caused by the role of *RAS* mutation in tumor dedifferentiation and progression to anaplastic carcinoma.[12] In a series of 91 tumors followed for a median of 14 years, *RAS* mutation correlated with distant metastasis and a significantly higher mortality.[56] Overall, because of its presence in benign and largely indolent tumors, the *RAS* mutation has not been a consistently reliable, prognostic biomarker.

Unlike PTCs with *BRAF* and *RAS* mutations, those with *RET/PTC* genetic rearrangement have shown a favorable prognosis.[57] They have been found to have a lower probability of tumor dedifferentiation and metastasis, but may be associated with a higher risk of lymph node involvement.

Genetic Analysis of Multifocal PTC

Multifocal PTC can represent either intraglandular spread from a single clonal cancer or multiple synchronous primary cancers. Using a series of 60 multifocal PTCs with 2 to 4 discrete tumor foci, genetic mutations, and histopathologic characteristics, we tested for *BRAF*, *NRAS*, *HRAS*, and *KRAS* point mutations and *RET/PTC1* and *RET/PTC3* rearrangements.[58] As expected, *BRAF* mutations were found in 43% of tumors, *RAS* in 27%, and *RET/PTC* in 2%. We identified 4 subgroups of these PTCs: (1) 2 foci containing different mutations (30%); (2) 1 tumor with a mutation and another without mutations (32%); (3) all cancers containing the same mutation (25%); and (4) absence of detectable mutations in all cancers (13%). We concluded that up to 60% of multifocal PTC were likely synchronous primary tumors because 30% of cases had 2 different mutations likely representing separate clonal cancers and, in an additional 30% of cases, one cancer had an identified mutation whereas the other did not. On histopathology, these multifocal cancers were also located in different lobes, showed distinct growth patterns, and showed no evidence of peritumoral dissemination.[58]

TECHNIQUES FOR BIOMARKER DETECTION

Testing for the various biomarkers is based on the type of mutation. For point mutations, *BRAF* and *RAS*, many different techniques have been shown to be effective: polymerase chain reaction (PCR) and Sanger sequencing, pyrosequencing, real-time PCR amplification with post-PCR melting curve analysis, and allele-specific PCR.[59]

In the Sanger method, the DNA strand to be analyzed is used as a template and a DNA polymerase is used to generate complimentary strands using primers. Four different PCR reaction mixtures are prepared, each containing a certain percentage of dideoxynucleoside triphosphate (ddNTP) analogues to one of the 4 nucleotides, which, when encountered during synthesis, terminates the reaction. Each of the 4 PCR reactions then has a mixture of different lengths of DNA strands, all ending with the nucleotide that was dideoxy labeled for that reaction. Gel electrophoresis is then used to separate the strands of the 4 reactions, in 4 separate lanes, and to determine the sequence of the original template based on what lengths of strands end with what nucleotide. The 4 reactions are then combined and applied to a single lane of a gel. Laser-generated chromatograms are then generated from which the template DNA sequence can be determined.

The pyrosequencing method allows sequencing of a single DNA by synthesizing the complementary strand 1 base pair at a time and detecting which base was added at each step. Solutions containing A, C, G, and T nucleotides are added sequentially and removed from the reaction. Light is produced only when the nucleotide solution complements the first unpaired base of the template, which results in chemiluminescent signals and elucidates the template sequence.

Real-time PCR quantifies the amount of a particular gene present by detecting fluorescence once double-stranded DNA is amplified. As the reaction proceeds, the point at which a certain threshold of fluorescence is reached indicates how much of the gene of interest is present in the sample.

In allele-specific PCR, a primer is chosen that contains the mutation in the gene of interest, which therefore only initiates the PCR reaction if the altered gene is present.

For the chromosomal rearrangements, *RET/PTC* and *PAX8/PPAR*γ, the testing can only be reliably performed on fresh or immediately frozen FNAB samples.[34] Reverse transcriptase PCR is used in either real-time mode or in a conventional fashion to detect the mutated RNA present. The sensitivity should not be too high, because the tissues acquire more chromosomal rearrangements as they age and become damaged. If testing samples fixed in formalin or paraffin, fluorescence in situ hybridization is the assay of choice because PCR is so sensitive. However, this makes testing on fixed tissue less practical in the clinical setting.

NGS

NGS offers simultaneous massively parallel sequencing of millions of DNA sequences and may be cost-effective for detecting multiple genetic alterations. An advantage compared with conventional Sanger sequencing is that it allows simultaneous analysis of large regions of the genome and offers high sensitivity of mutation detection and quantitative assessment of mutant alleles. NGS comprises whole-genome sequencing, whole-exome sequencing, and whole-transcriptome sequencing as well as targeted sequencing of multiple specific genomic regions. Targeted NGS panels may improve routine molecular diagnostics of cancer. In thyroid nodules, such an approach may be helpful to expand the currently available diagnostic panels of several genes to enable simultaneous testing for multiple mutations. Our group recently evaluated targeted next-generation sequencing as a new approach for testing a broader spectrum of point mutations that occur in thyroid cancer.[60] Among FTCs, somatic *TSHR* mutations were identified in 22% of cases. Of 7 *TSHR* mutations identified, 5 were in malignant and 2 in benign nodules, suggesting that the location of this mutation in a thyroid nodule may have some association with thyroid cancer, particularly with follicular carcinoma. Another significant observation was the detection of *TP53* mutations in oncocytic follicular carcinomas. *TP53* mutations are known to occur with increasing frequency in dedifferentiating thyroid tumors but not in well-differentiated cancer. The high frequency of *TP53* mutations in these tumors was not caused by a sensitive detection using the NGS approach because the mutation was found at high allelic frequency. However, *TP53* mutation occurred in approximately 20% of oncocytic follicular cancers, suggesting that this tumor subset may be prone to dedifferentiation, providing a potential diagnostic and prognostic marker in this cancer type.

The high frequency of mutation detection in thyroid cancers by ThyroSeq is expected to further improve the sensitivity of cancer detection in thyroid nodules with indeterminate FNA cytology that are currently tested using more limited mutational panels. Because of the inclusion of additional gene hotspots such as within *TP53* and *TSHR*, as many as 68% of all tumor types were identified by the ThyroSeq panel to carry at least one point mutation. If combined with the detection of chromosomal rearrangements, potentially more than 80% of all thyroid cancer would be expected to have at least one detectable mutational event. Extended mutational profiling using the ThyroSeq panel revealed that 9 of 99 mutation-positive cancers (9%) contained more than one mutation. These tumors included either dedifferentiated tumors (6 anaplastic and 1 PDTC) or PTCs (n = 2), both with unfavorable prognostic features such as distant metastasis or local tumor recurrence. Most of these tumors had a combination of either *BRAF* or *NRAS* mutation, known to be an early driver event in thyroid cancer, and *TP53* and/or *PIK3CA* mutation, which are thought to be late events in tumor clone progression. The occurrence of multiple mutations has been reported before in advanced thyroid cancer and was observed in this study, suggesting that, in addition to its diagnostic utility, this comprehensive mutational panel may further contribute to preoperative thyroid cancer risk stratification by mutation testing of FNAB samples.

SUMMARY

Molecular techniques to detect mutations and rearrangements in thyroid FNAB specimens has already shown significant clinical utility in improving the preoperative diagnosis of well-differentiated thyroid carcinomas, and has been particularly useful for risk stratification of cytologically indeterminate FNAB results. With emerging new technologies that continue to broaden the spectrum of evaluable genetic alterations, the accessibility and applicability of molecular testing is likely to continue to expand. The added preoperative prognostic information can also be used to help guide extent of initial surgery, although future study is still needed to determine whether tailored operative management will improve disease outcomes.

REFERENCES

1. SEER Cancer Statistics Review [Internet]. National Cancer Institute. 1975-2005. Available at: http://seer.cancer.gov/csr/1975_2005/. Accessed December 1, 2013.
2. Mazzaferri EL. Management of a solitary thyroid nodule. N Engl J Med 1993; 328(8):553–9.

3. American Thyroid Association Guidelines Taskforce on Thyroid Nodules, Differentiated Thyroid Cancer, Cooper DS, Doherty GM, Haugen BR, et al. Revised American Thyroid Association management guidelines for patients with thyroid nodules and differentiated thyroid cancer. Thyroid 2009;19(11):1167–214.
4. Gharib H, Papini E, Paschke R, et al. American Association of Clinical Endocrinologists, Associazione Medici Endocrinologi, and European Thyroid Association medical guidelines for clinical practice for the diagnosis and management of thyroid nodules: executive summary of recommendations. J Endocrinol Invest 2010; 33(Suppl 5):51–6.
5. Mehta V, Nikiforov YE, Ferris RL. Use of molecular biomarkers in FNA specimens to personalize treatment for thyroid surgery. Head Neck 2013;35(10):1499–506.
6. Hamberger B, Gharib H, Melton LJ 3rd, et al. Fine-needle aspiration biopsy of thyroid nodules. Impact on thyroid practice and cost of care. Am J Med 1982; 73(3):381–4.
7. Wang CC, Friedman L, Kennedy GC, et al. A large multicenter correlation study of thyroid nodule cytopathology and histopathology. Thyroid 2011;21(3): 243–51.
8. Bongiovanni M, Spitale A, Faquin WC, et al. The Bethesda System for Reporting Thyroid Cytopathology: a meta-analysis. Acta Cytol 2012;56(4):333–9.
9. Baloch ZW, LiVolsi VA, Asa SL, et al. Diagnostic terminology and morphologic criteria for cytologic diagnosis of thyroid lesions: a synopsis of the National Cancer Institute Thyroid Fine-Needle Aspiration State of the Science Conference. Diagn Cytopathol 2008;36(6):425–37.
10. Chen JC, Pace SC, Chen BA, et al. Yield of repeat fine-needle aspiration biopsy and rate of malignancy in patients with atypia or follicular lesion of undetermined significance: the impact of the Bethesda System for Reporting Thyroid Cytopathology. Surgery 2012;152(6):1037–44.
11. Heller M, Zanocco K, Zydowicz S, et al. Cost-effectiveness analysis of repeat fine-needle aspiration for thyroid biopsies read as atypia of undetermined significance. Surgery 2012;152(3):423–30.
12. Nikiforov YE, Nikiforova MN. Molecular genetics and diagnosis of thyroid cancer. Nat Rev Endocrinol 2011;7(10):569–80.
13. Xing M. Molecular pathogenesis and mechanisms of thyroid cancer. Nat Rev Cancer 2013;13(3):184–99.
14. Nikiforova MN, Nikiforov YE. Molecular diagnostics and predictors in thyroid cancer. Thyroid 2009;19(12):1351–61.
15. Chakravarty D, Santos E, Ryder M, et al. Small-molecule MAPK inhibitors restore radioiodine incorporation in mouse thyroid cancers with conditional BRAF activation. J Clin Invest 2011;121(12):4700–11.
16. Nehs MA, Nucera C, Nagarkatti SS, et al. Late intervention with anti-BRAF(V600E) therapy induces tumor regression in an orthotopic mouse model of human anaplastic thyroid cancer. Endocrinology 2012;153(2):985–94.
17. Lee ST, Kim SW, Ki CS, et al. Clinical implication of highly sensitive detection of the BRAF V600E mutation in fine-needle aspirations of thyroid nodules: a comparative analysis of three molecular assays in 4585 consecutive cases in a BRAF V600E mutation-prevalent area. J Clin Endocrinol Metab 2012;97(7): 2299–306.
18. Ohori NP, Singhal R, Nikiforova MN, et al. BRAF mutation detection in indeterminate thyroid cytology specimens: underlying cytologic, molecular, and pathologic characteristics of papillary thyroid carcinoma. Cancer Cytopathol 2013; 121(4):197–205.

19. Howell GM, Hodak SP, Yip L. RAS mutations in thyroid cancer. Oncologist 2013; 18(8):926–32.
20. Tallini G, Asa SL. RET oncogene activation in papillary thyroid carcinoma. Adv Anat Pathol 2001;8(6):345–54.
21. Nikiforov YE. RET/PTC rearrangement in thyroid tumors. Endocr Pathol 2002; 13(1):3–16.
22. Nikiforov YE, Rowland JM, Bove KE, et al. Distinct pattern of ret oncogene rearrangements in morphological variants of radiation-induced and sporadic thyroid papillary carcinomas in children. Cancer Res 1997;57(9):1690–4.
23. Rabes HM, Demidchik EP, Sidorow JD, et al. Pattern of radiation-induced RET and NTRK1 rearrangements in 191 post-Chernobyl papillary thyroid carcinomas: biological, phenotypic, and clinical implications. Clin Cancer Res 2000;6(3):1093–103.
24. Fenton CL, Lukes Y, Nicholson D, et al. The ret/PTC mutations are common in sporadic papillary thyroid carcinoma of children and young adults. J Clin Endocrinol Metab 2000;85(3):1170–5.
25. Adeniran AJ, Zhu Z, Gandhi M, et al. Correlation between genetic alterations and microscopic features, clinical manifestations, and prognostic characteristics of thyroid papillary carcinomas. Am J Surg Pathol 2006;30(2):216–22.
26. Elisei R, Romei C, Vorontsova T, et al. RET/PTC rearrangements in thyroid nodules: studies in irradiated and not irradiated, malignant and benign thyroid lesions in children and adults. J Clin Endocrinol Metab 2001;86(7):3211–6.
27. Saji M, Ringel MD. The PI3K-Akt-mTOR pathway in initiation and progression of thyroid tumors. Mol Cell Endocrinol 2010;321(1):20–8.
28. Ringel MD, Hayre N, Saito J, et al. Overexpression and overactivation of Akt in thyroid carcinoma. Cancer Res 2001;61(16):6105–11.
29. Kroll TG, Sarraf P, Pęcciarini L, et al. PAX8-PPARgamma1 fusion oncogene in human thyroid carcinoma [corrected]. Science 2000;289(5483):1357–60.
30. Eberhardt NL, Grebe SK, McIver B, et al. The role of the PAX8/PPARgamma fusion oncogene in the pathogenesis of follicular thyroid cancer. Mol Cell Endocrinol 2010;321(1):50–6.
31. McIver B, Grebe SK, Eberhardt NL. The PAX8/PPAR gamma fusion oncogene as a potential therapeutic target in follicular thyroid carcinoma. Curr Drug Targets Immune Endocr Metabol Disord 2004;4(3):221–34.
32. Nikiforova MN, Lynch RA, Biddinger PW, et al. RAS point mutations and PAX8-PPAR gamma rearrangement in thyroid tumors: evidence for distinct molecular pathways in thyroid follicular carcinoma. J Clin Endocrinol Metab 2003;88(5):2318–26.
33. Garcia-Rostan G, Zhao H, Camp RL, et al. ras mutations are associated with aggressive tumor phenotypes and poor prognosis in thyroid cancer. J Clin Oncol 2003;21(17):3226–35.
34. Nikiforov YE, Ohori NP, Hodak SP, et al. Impact of mutational testing on the diagnosis and management of patients with cytologically indeterminate thyroid nodules: a prospective analysis of 1056 FNA samples. J Clin Endocrinol Metab 2011;96(11):3390–7.
35. Gupta N, Dasyam AK, Carty SE, et al. RAS mutations in thyroid FNA specimens are highly predictive of predominantly low-risk follicular-pattern cancers. J Clin Endocrinol Metab 2013;98(5):E914–22.
36. Mathur A, Weng J, Moses W, et al. A prospective study evaluating the accuracy of using combined clinical factors and candidate diagnostic markers to refine the accuracy of thyroid fine needle aspiration biopsy. Surgery 2010;148(6): 1170–6 [discussion: 1176–7].

37. Cheung CC, Carydis B, Ezzat S, et al. Analysis of ret/PTC gene rearrangements refines the fine needle aspiration diagnosis of thyroid cancer. J Clin Endocrinol Metab 2001;86(5):2187–90.
38. Cantara S, Capezzone M, Marchisotta S, et al. Impact of proto-oncogene mutation detection in cytological specimens from thyroid nodules improves the diagnostic accuracy of cytology. J Clin Endocrinol Metab 2010;95(3):1365–9.
39. Nikiforov YE, Steward DL, Robinson-Smith TM, et al. Molecular testing for mutations in improving the fine-needle aspiration diagnosis of thyroid nodules. J Clin Endocrinol Metab 2009;94(6):2092–8.
40. Yip L, WL, Armstrong MJ, et al. A clinical algorithm for fine-needle aspiration molecular testing effectively guides the appropriate extent of initial thyroidectomy. Ann Surg, in press.
41. Yip L, Farris C, Kabaker AS, et al. Cost impact of molecular testing for indeterminate thyroid nodule fine-needle aspiration biopsies. J Clin Endocrinol Metab 2012;97(6):1905–12.
42. Mehta RS, Carty SE, Ohori NP, et al. Nodule size is an independent predictor of malignancy in mutation-negative nodules with follicular lesion of undetermined significance cytology. Surgery 2013;154(4):730–6 [discussion: 736–8].
43. Xing M. BRAF mutation in papillary thyroid cancer: pathogenic role, molecular bases, and clinical implications. Endocr Rev 2007;28(7):742–62.
44. Elisei R, Ugolini C, Viola D, et al. BRAF(V600E) mutation and outcome of patients with papillary thyroid carcinoma: a 15-year median follow-up study. J Clin Endocrinol Metab 2008;93(10):3943–9.
45. Xing M, Alzahrani AS, Carson KA, et al. Association between BRAF V600E mutation and mortality in patients with papillary thyroid cancer. JAMA 2013;309(14):1493–501.
46. American Thyroid Association Surgery Working Group, American Association of Endocrine Surgeons, American Academy of Otolaryngology-Head and Neck Surgery, American Head and Neck Society, Carty SE, Cooper DS, Doherty GM, et al. Consensus statement on the terminology and classification of central neck dissection for thyroid cancer. Thyroid 2009;19(11):1153–8.
47. Hughes DT, White ML, Miller BS, et al. Influence of prophylactic central lymph node dissection on postoperative thyroglobulin levels and radioiodine treatment in papillary thyroid cancer. Surgery 2010;148(6):1100–6 [discussion: 1006–7].
48. Popadich A, Levin O, Lee JC, et al. A multicenter cohort study of total thyroidectomy and routine central lymph node dissection for cN0 papillary thyroid cancer. Surgery 2011;150(6):1048–57.
49. Wang TS, Cheung K, Farrokhyar F, et al. A meta-analysis of the effect of prophylactic central compartment neck dissection on locoregional recurrence rates in patients with papillary thyroid cancer. Ann Surg Oncol 2013;20(11):3477–83.
50. Lang BH, Wong KP, Wan KY, et al. Impact of routine unilateral central neck dissection on preablative and postablative stimulated thyroglobulin levels after total thyroidectomy in papillary thyroid carcinoma. Ann Surg Oncol 2012;19(1):60–7.
51. Howell GM, Nikiforova MN, Carty SE, et al. BRAF V600E mutation independently predicts central compartment lymph node metastasis in patients with papillary thyroid cancer. Ann Surg Oncol 2013;20(1):47–52.
52. Lee KC, Li C, Schneider EB, et al. Is BRAF mutation associated with lymph node metastasis in patients with papillary thyroid cancer? Surgery 2012;152(6):977–83.

53. Rodolico V, Cabibi D, Pizzolanti G, et al. BRAF V600E mutation and p27 kip1 expression in papillary carcinomas of the thyroid $\leq$1 cm and their paired lymph node metastases. Cancer 2007;110(6):1218–26.
54. Lupi C, Giannini R, Ugolini C, et al. Association of BRAF V600E mutation with poor clinicopathological outcomes in 500 consecutive cases of papillary thyroid carcinoma. J Clin Endocrinol Metab 2007;92(11):4085–90.
55. Niemeier LA, Kuffner Akatsu H, Song C, et al. A combined molecular-pathologic score improves risk stratification of thyroid papillary microcarcinoma. Cancer 2012;118(8):2069–77.
56. Hara H, Fulton N, Yashiro T, et al. N-ras mutation: an independent prognostic factor for aggressiveness of papillary thyroid carcinoma. Surgery 1994;116(6): 1010–6.
57. Soares P, Fonseca E, Wynford-Thomas D, et al. Sporadic ret-rearranged papillary carcinoma of the thyroid: a subset of slow growing, less aggressive thyroid neoplasms? J Pathol 1998;185(1):71–8.
58. Bansal M, Gandhi M, Ferris RL, et al. Molecular and histopathologic characteristics of multifocal papillary thyroid carcinoma. Am J Surg Pathol 2013;37(10): 1586–91.
59. Jin L, Sebo TJ, Nakamura N, et al. BRAF mutation analysis in fine needle aspiration (FNA) cytology of the thyroid. Diagn Mol Pathol 2006;15(3):136–43.
60. Nikiforova MN, Wald AI, Roy S, et al. Targeted next-generation sequencing panel (ThyroSeq) for detection of mutations in thyroid cancer. J Clin Endocrinol Metab 2013;98(11):E1852–60.

Clinical Diagnostic Gene Expression Thyroid Testing

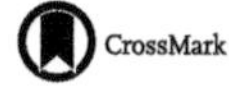

David L. Steward, MD[a,b], Richard T. Kloos, MD[c,*]

KEYWORDS

- Biopsy • Fine-needle aspirate • Gene expression • Genomics
- Molecular diagnostic techniques • DNA mutational analysis • Thyroid nodule

KEY POINTS

- Fifteen to 30% of thyroid fine-needle aspiration biopsies are cytologically indeterminate.
- When cytologically indeterminate thyroid nodules undergo diagnostic surgery, approximately three-quarters prove to be benign.
- The Afirma Gene Expression Classifier (GEC) achieved a risk of malignancy of 6% or less on an independent set of 265 prospectively collected cytologically indeterminate nodules when the molecular results were compared with the blinded gold standard central expert histopathology diagnosis.
- The National Comprehensive Cancer Network Thyroid Carcinoma Guideline states that cytologically indeterminate thyroid nodules determined to have a malignancy risk of ~5% or less with a molecular test can be clinically observed.
- For GEC-tested patients, published clinical utility studies demonstrate that approximately half of those with indeterminate cytology (Bethesda III/IV) avoid diagnostic thyroid surgery.

THYROID CANCER MULTIGENE EXPRESSION CLASSIFIERS: WHAT THE SURGEON SHOULD KNOW

Introduction

Before the advent of thyroid nodule fine-needle aspiration biopsy (FNAB), thyroid nodules were routinely referred for diagnostic surgery because of their 5% to 15% risk of malignancy (ROM).[1] FNAB decreased diagnostic thyroidectomies by one-half

Disclosure Statement: R.T. Kloos is a stock option holder and employee of Veracyte, Inc. The opinions expressed are those of the authors and may not reflect the opinions of Veracyte. D.L. Steward has received research funding from Veracyte as part of published clinical trials.
[a] Department of Otolaryngology–Head and Neck Surgery, University of Cincinnati College of Medicine, 231 Albert Sabin Way, Cincinnati, OH 45267-0528, USA; [b] Division of Endocrinology, Department of Medicine, University of Cincinnati College of Medicine, 231 Albert Sabin Way, Cincinnati, OH 45267-0528, USA; [c] Department of Medical Affairs, Veracyte, Inc, 7000 Shoreline Court, Suite 250, South San Francisco, CA 94080, USA
* Corresponding author.
E-mail address: Richard.Kloos@veracyte.com

Otolaryngol Clin N Am 47 (2014) 573–593
http://dx.doi.org/10.1016/j.otc.2014.04.009
oto.theclinics.com

because most FNABs are diagnosed as cytologically benign.[2] Still, 15% to 30% of thyroid FNABs are cytologically indeterminate (ie, not clearly benign nor malignant).[1,3] When cytologically indeterminate thyroid nodules undergo diagnostic surgery, approximately three-quarters prove to be histologically benign.[4,5] Therefore, patient care could be significantly improved with genomic diagnostic technologies that accurately reclassify these samples as benign with high enough negative predictive value (NPV) to safely avoid the costs and risks of diagnostic thyroid surgery. In choosing which genomic test to order, the surgeon should insure that peer-reviewed publications exist that define the test's clinical and analytical validity, and most importantly, its clinical utility.

Currently, the Afirma gene expression classifier (GEC) (Veracyte Inc, South San Francisco, CA, USA) is used in cytologically indeterminate nodules (Bethesda III and IV) to reclassify them as benign nodules and to avoid diagnostic surgery. **Table 1** lists the Bethesda cytologic category definitions. By accurately excluding malignancy when the test result is benign, the Afirma GEC is known as a "rule-out" test.[6] In addition, it identifies rare neoplasms that are often difficult to diagnose accurately with cytology, such as medullary thyroid cancer (MTC), parathyroid neoplasms, and certain metastases to the thyroid. Given the wealth of published data regarding the Afirma GEC's clinical validity,[7,8] analytical validity,[9] and clinical utility,[10,11] patients should not undergo thyroid surgery for solely diagnostic reasons for lower risk cytologically indeterminate thyroid nodules (Bethesda III and IV) without the physician and patient considering the role of Afirma GEC testing. In the surgical author's practice, approximately half of the patients with cytologically indeterminate nodules chose to pursue surgery over additional testing. Younger patients, and those with a higher ROM based on cytology (Bethesda V vs Bethesda III/IV), were more likely to elect surgery.[12] For those who chose GEC testing, half avoided thyroid surgery, similar to what was found in 2 multicenter clinical utility studies of Afirma.[10,11]

Cost, Morbidity, and Risk of Mortality from Surgery

The average direct costs of hemithyroidectomy and total thyroidectomy are conservatively estimated at greater than $6000 and $11,000, respectively.[13] However, the range of costs for these procedures at various inpatient facilities exceeds $20,000 and $25,000, respectively.[13] Nevertheless, the costs of diagnostic surgery include more than just the direct cost of the procedure. Estimates of costs of diagnostic thyroidectomy should include surgical complications, as well as indirect costs due to time lost from work and responsibilities of daily living (eg, child care, cooking, cleaning), impaired quality of life (the fear of potentially having cancer and the anxiety of undergoing diagnostic surgery, postoperative pain and recovery, and the potentially impaired quality of life from iatrogenic hypothyroidism with,[14] or without,[15] a normal serum TSH).

Although thyroid lobectomy is increasingly performed as an outpatient procedure with excellent outcomes in experienced hands, the outcomes from thyroidectomy overall can be sobering. Thyroid surgery is associated with a perioperative mortality of 0.1% to 0.2%, with rates as high as 0.5%.[16–18] Serious or permanent nonlethal complications of thyroidectomy include hypocalcemia, recurrent and/or superior laryngeal nerve damage, rebleeding, and wound infection.[19,20] The frequency of these complications is underappreciated and is strongly related to surgeon experience (volume) and expertise. One study reported that 11% of patients undergoing thyroidectomy or parathyroidectomy required a visit to the emergency room at least once within 30 days of surgery, and nearly one-quarter of these patients required hospitalization.[21] Complication rates from thyroid surgery may be much higher in

Table 1
Performance of the Afirma GEC

GEC result	Malignant reference standard	Benign reference standard	
Bethesda Categories III–V (n = 265)			
GEC result	Malignant reference standard (n = 85)	Benign reference standard (n = 180)	Sensitivity, 92% [84–97]
			Specificity, 52% [44–59]
Suspicious	78	87	PPV, 47% [40–55]
Benign	7	93	NPV, 93% [86–97]
			%FN results, 2.6%
			ROM, 32%
Bethesda Category III: Atypia of undetermined significance/Follicular lesion of undetermined significance (n = 129)			
GEC result	Malignant reference standard (n = 31)	Benign reference standard (n = 98)	Sensitivity, 90% [74–98]
			Specificity, 53% [43–63]
Suspicious	28	46	PPV, 38% [27–50]
Benign	3	52	NPV, 95% [85–99]
			%FN results, 2.3%
			ROM, 24%
Bethesda Category IV: Follicular or Hürthle cell neoplasm/Suspicious for follicular neoplasm (FN/SFN) (n = 81)			
GEC result	Malignant reference standard (n = 20)	Benign reference standard (n = 61)	Sensitivity, 90% [68–99]
			Specificity, 49% [36–62]
Suspicious	18	31	PPV, 37% [23–52]
Benign	2	30	NPV, 94% [79–99]
			%FN results, 2.5%
			ROM, 25%
Bethesda Category V: Suspicious for malignancy (n = 55)			
GEC result	Malignant reference standard (n = 34)	Benign reference standard (n = 21)	Sensitivity, 94% [80–99]
			Specificity, 52% [30–74]
Suspicious	32	10	PPV, 76% [61–88]
Benign	2	11	NPV, 85% [55–98]
			%FN results, 3.6%
			ROM, 62%
Bethesda Category II: Cytopathology benign (n = 47)			
GEC result	Malignant reference standard (n = 3)	Benign reference standard (n = 44)	Sensitivity, 100% [29–100]
			Specificity, 70% [55–83]
Suspicious	3	13	PPV, 19% [5–46]
Benign	0	31	NPV, 100% [86–100]
			%FN results, 0%
			ROM, 6%

Abbreviations: ROM, risk of malignancy (malignancy prevalence); %FN, percentage false negative.

Adapted from Alexander EK, Kennedy GC, Baloch ZW, et al. Preoperative diagnosis of benign thyroid nodules with indeterminate cytology. N Engl J Med 2012;367(8):710.

population-based series than in high-volume single academic center series. For example, complications in the state of Maryland were found to be 10.1% for surgeons who did between 1 and 9 cases per year, and 5.9% for surgeons who did more than one hundred cases per year.[22] In fact, more than 50% of thyroid surgeries in the United States are performed by surgeons who do 5 or fewer cases per year,[23] placing many patients at increased risk of complications.

Given the costs and potential complications of diagnostic surgery, efforts to avoid unnecessary surgery are in the best interests of the patient, the health care system, and the physician.

Regulation of Molecular Diagnostic Tests

Laboratory developed tests are currently regulated by the Clinical Laboratory Improvement Amendments (CLIA). Congress passed CLIA in 1988 to establish quality standards for all laboratory testing to ensure the accuracy, reliability, and timeliness of patient test results, regardless of where the test was performed.

In 2004, the Office of Public Health Genomics (OPHG) of the Centers for Disease Control and Prevention (CDC) recognized a critical need for providing guidance to health care providers and patients on the appropriate use of the genomic tests. In response, the OPHG launched Evaluation of Genomic Applications in Practice and Prevention (EGAPP), the first federal evidence-based initiative to address genomic testing specifically.[24] The EGAPP Working Group was established by the National Office of Public Health Genomics at the CDC to standardize evaluation of the rapidly emerging array of genomics diagnostic tests. EGAPP adapts existing evidence review methods to the systematic evaluation of genomic tests and links scientific evidence to clinical recommendations for the use of genomic tests.

In 2009, EGAPP developed a set of methods based on the evaluation of analytical validity, clinical validity, clinical utility, and, to some extent, the ethical, legal, and social implications of each test.[24] Analytic validity includes analytic sensitivity (detection rate of a known positive), analytic specificity (1 − false positive rate), reliability (eg, repeatability of test results), and assay robustness (eg, resistance to small changes in preanalytic or analytic variables such as reagent variability or interfering substances).[25] EGAPP defines the clinical validity of a genetic test as its ability to predict accurately and reliably the clinically defined disorder or phenotype of interest (eg, benign vs malignant nodule).[25] Clinical validity encompasses clinical sensitivity and specificity, and predictive values of positive and negative tests that take into account the disorder prevalence.[25] Finally, the clinical utility of a genetic test is the evidence of improved measurable clinical outcomes, and its usefulness and added value to patient management decision-making compared with current management without genetic testing.[25] For example, a test can have excellent analytical and clinical validity, but if patient outcome is not improved, then clinical utility is not established.

Unfortunately, most physicians and specialty societies do not rigorously evaluate tests as proposed by EGAPP. They often assume that if the test is available, then analytic and clinical validity, as well as clinical utility, have been established. Unfortunately, most suppliers of genomic tests fail to perform robust analytical validation studies or the clinical utility studies necessary to demonstrate improved health care outcomes. Insurance company payers regard clinical utility studies as a key determinant of whether a test is medically necessary and deny paying for new genomic tests because of the lack of demonstrated clinical utility for more than any other reason.[26] Of the commercially available products for molecular testing of thyroid nodules, only the Afirma GEC has published evidence of analytical validity, clinical validity, and clinical utility (**Fig. 1**),[27] which has resulted in widespread payer coverage for the Afirma GEC.

Veracyte Afirma GEC

The Afirma GEC is based on the measurement of messenger RNA (mRNA) expression. There are 2 key advantages to using RNA instead of DNA for test development. First, although there are only approximately 23,000 known protein-coding DNA genes,[28] each of these may be transcribed into multiple alternatively spliced variants, with more than 240,000 known mRNA isoforms. Disease-causing alterations in the DNA generally exert their effects, at least partially, on the transcriptome. Therefore, mRNA transcript measurement provides an amplification of the effects caused by

Test	Published Clinical Validity in Cytologically Indeterminate Samples			Published Analytical Validity	Published Clinical Utility[a]
	Sensitivity	NPV	Blinded gold standard histopathology		
Afirma® GEC	90%	≥94%	✓	✓	✓
Mutation Panel (UPMC)	59%	90%	X	✓	X
Mutation Panel (Asuragen, Quest, LabCorp)	X	X	X	X	X
Mutation Panel + miRNA expression (Asuragen)	X	X	X	X	X
Mutation Panel (ThyroSeq)	X	X	X	✓	X

Fig. 1. Published results for Bethesda III/IV FNAB molecular diagnostics. Clinical validity requires performance characteristics in the intended use samples (eg, Bethesda III and IV cytology specimens). The EGAPP Working Group developed a set of methods based on the evaluation of analytical validity, clinical validity, clinical utility, and, to some extent, the ethical, legal, and social implications of each test.[24] [a] Clinical utility here refers to the decision to elect clinical observation of the nodule in lieu of diagnostic surgery. (*Data from* Refs.[7,29,69])

upstream changes in the DNA blueprint that are quite a bit more difficult to identify without large-scale de novo sequencing. Second, gene expression may be impacted by lifestyle and environmental factors so mRNA gene expression reflects additional information not discernible from DNA analysis alone. The quantification of mRNA expression captures upstream DNA point mutations and gene rearrangements, as well as the actions of microRNAs, which may regulate gene expression. This approach avoids the limitation that common DNA mutations are not present in many cytologically indeterminate nodules. In fact, the most common DNA mutations are so low in frequency in Bethesda III/IV nodules that 7 individuals must be tested to obtain one gene mutation–positive result.[29] Similarly, benign thyroid nodules may carry DNA mutations. Transcriptional analysis assists in identifying gene signatures that reflect whole patterns of pathway activation versus analysis of a small number of genes.[30]

The GEC was developed and validated clinically to identify preoperatively histologically benign nodules among those with indeterminate cytology. Instead of relying on genes previously identified in the literature, analysis of the whole genome (transcriptome) was used to identify candidate genes, and support vector machine learning methods were used to develop the classifier algorithm.[7,8] By preoperatively identifying patients with cytologically indeterminate nodules who are at low risk of having cancer, clinical and sonographic follow-up may be recommended in lieu of diagnostic surgery, thus ending the diagnostic odyssey (**Fig. 2**).[31,32] This approach answers the question of whether one should operate or observe an indeterminate nodule, as opposed to "rule-in" tests, which may be used to answer the question of whether a total versus hemithyroidectomy should be performed. Gene mutation testing and gene expression profiles have been developed to answer the latter question.[6,33,34] The Afirma GEC

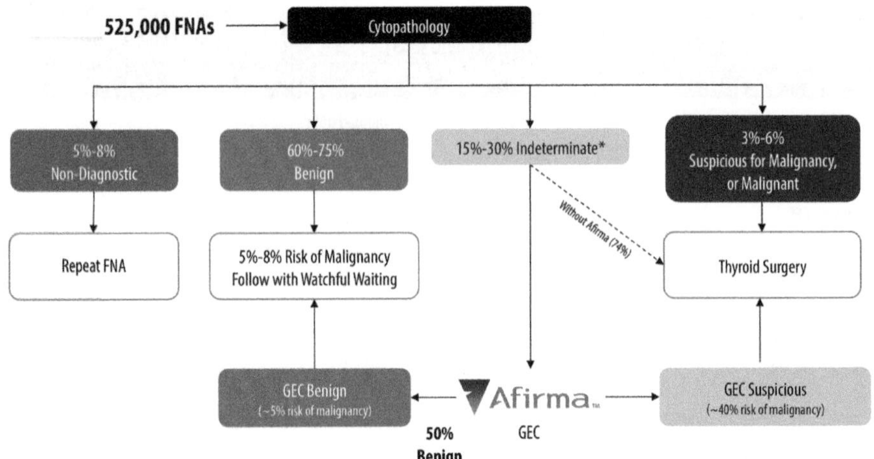

Fig. 2. Implementing the Afirma GEC into clinical practice. *Cytologically indeterminate nodules are Bethesda categories III and IV.[73] (*Data from* Refs.[1,8,10,38,70–72])

analysis is indicated only for nodules with indeterminate cytology and is not performed on cytologically benign, malignant, or nondiagnostic (insufficient) FNAB samples.

The Afirma GEC test is performed in Veracyte's CLIA-certified clinical laboratory. The molecular classifier proceeds in a stepwise fashion, first applying 6 cassettes before applying the final benign versus malignant classifier. These cassettes differentiate specific uncommon neoplasm subtypes that are often missed by cytology and act as filters that halt further sample processing if any cassette returns a "suspicious" result. These cassettes classify samples representing (1) malignant melanoma, (2) renal cell carcinoma, (3) breast carcinoma, (4) parathyroid tissue, and (5) medullary thyroid carcinoma. A final cassette (6) was also trained using Hürthle cell adenomas and carcinomas to identify Hürthle cell neoplasms versus Hürthle cell changes or features related to thyroiditis or hyperplasia. Failing to trigger one of these cassettes, the GEC evaluates the expression of 142 genes that are used in a proprietary mathematical algorithm to classify indeterminate thyroid nodule FNABs as either "benign" or "suspicious." The genes used in the cassettes and main GEC classifier are published.[7]

Analytical Validity

The GEC performance was evaluated in a series of 43 individual reagent and analytical verification studies.[9] Extensive reagent and analytical performance studies were conducted to evaluate the reliability and reproducibility of the GEC under a variety of experimental and clinical conditions, with robust and highly reproducible results.[9] Interfering substances, including human blood and genomic DNA, were not found to interfere with extraction or amplification steps of the assay. Analytical sensitivity studies demonstrated tolerance to variations in RNA input across the range of 5 ng to 25 ng, as well as to dilution of malignant FNAB material down to 20% with FNAB material from lymphocytic thyroiditis and nodule hyperplasia.[8,9] Analytical sensitivity and specificity studies with blood (up to 83%) and genomic DNA (30%) demonstrated negligible assay interference, although false positive results could result from very bloody FNABs.[9] FNAB preservative solution maintained high quality and quantity of RNA material under various stressed time, temperature, and shipping conditions with no significant effect on GEC scores, or "benign" versus "suspicious" calls

(100% concordance).[9] Based on these data, room-temperature storage at the clinical site and chilled-box shipping were verified for routine practice.

Clinical Validity and Clinical Practice Experience

The initial clinical validation publication of the Afirma GEC was performed on an independent sample set of cytologically indeterminate thyroid nodule FNABs within a prospective multicenter, double-blind study design.[8] The Afirma GEC achieved high sensitivity and NPV. After further optimization, the GEC was validated in a second larger independent sample set in a prospective multicenter validation study. Using independent test sets is essential to demonstrating that the GEC algorithm is not overtrained. The second study included the largest ever prospectively collected set of thyroid FNAB biopsies from 3789 unique patients. Based on the expected 24% prevalence of malignancy in cytologically indeterminate samples in clinical practice, a 95% NPV for the Afirma GEC was achieved on an independent sample set of 265 cytologically indeterminate nodules when the molecular results were compared with blinded gold standard central expert histopathology diagnosis.[7]

Analysis of atypia of undetermined significance versus follicular lesion of undetermined significance samples, both of which are Bethesda category III lesions, found no difference in sensitivity or specificity (RT Kloos, unpublished data, 2013). Overall, the ROM for a thyroid nodule with Bethesda categories III and IV indeterminate cytology with an Afirma GEC Benign classifier result is about 5% (see **Table 1**). This risk is comparable to the 6% to 8% cancer risk for an operated thyroid nodule with a benign cytology diagnosis (see **Fig. 2**; **Fig. 3**, see **Table 1**),[4,7,35–39] which demonstrates that cytologically indeterminate nodules (Bethesda categories III and IV) with an Afirma GEC benign diagnosis can be managed as would a cytologically benign

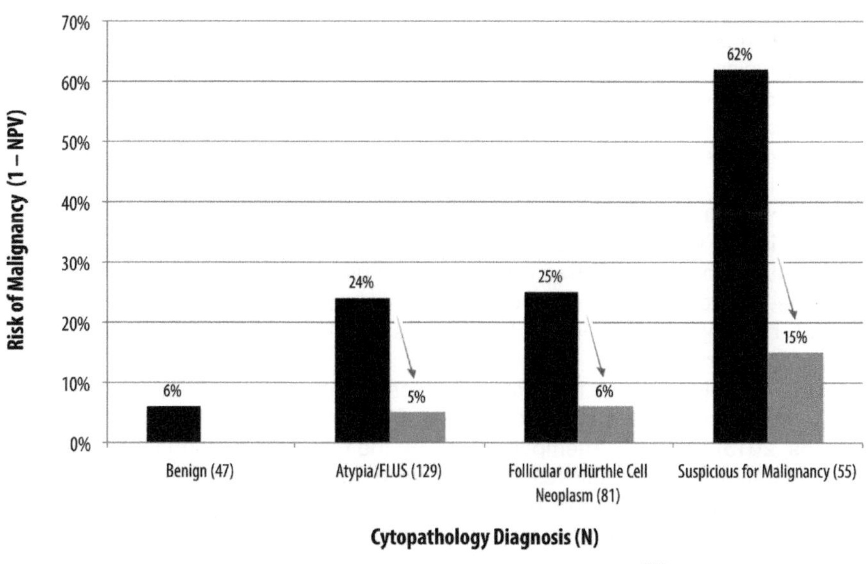

Fig. 3. Afirma GEC reclassifies cytologically indeterminate thyroid nodules with a benign genomic signature to GEC benign.[7] ROM is 1 – NPV. (*Adapted from* Alexander EK, Kennedy GC, Baloch ZW, et al. Preoperative diagnosis of benign thyroid nodules with indeterminate cytology. N Engl J Med 2012;367(8):705–15.)

nodule, as suggested by the National Comprehensive Cancer Network Thyroid Carcinoma Guideline.[32]

Unlike sensitivity and specificity, which are unaffected by the prevalence of cancer, positive predictive values (PPV) and NPV are influenced by the ROM in the cohort being evaluated. This influence complicates comparing the NPVs of different tests when they are described on different cohorts with different prevalences of cancer. One statistic to simplify such a comparison is the likelihood ratio. The formula for the likelihood ratio of a negative test (LR−) is (1 − sensitivity)/specificity.[40] The result should be between 0 and 1. A result of 1 indicates that the result is just as likely in those with the disease as in those without the disease, and it adds no value. Conversely, the test closest to 0 has the greater resolving power to exclude a condition. For the GEC, the likelihood ratio of a negative test in Bethesda III + IV is 0.19,[7] whereas the comparable LR− of mutational markers reported by Nikiforov and colleagues[29] is 0.42.

Specificity is the percentage of truly benign nodules identified by the test as benign. Cytologically indeterminate thyroid nodules have 0% specificity because they are not identified as benign with the microscope. Thus, the GEC raises the pretest specificity from 0% for cytologically indeterminate categories to 52% posttest, indicating that over half of the benign nodules from Bethesda categories III and IV can be identified and removed from the surgical pool. The sensitivity and specificity performance of the GEC were comparable across Bethesda III–V cytologies (see **Table 1**). However, given the higher prevalence of malignancy in Bethesda category V nodules (suspicious for malignancy), the NPV is lowered to 85% (see **Fig. 3**, **Table 1**). Thus, although the ROM is reduced from an initial 62% based on the cytologic category to 15% when the GEC is benign, surgery may not be avoidable based on the residual ROM. These Bethesda V nodules are therefore not routinely tested with the GEC. However, some physicians specifically request the GEC be performed in this cytologic category to screen the sample for rare neoplasms, such as medullary thyroid carcinoma.[41,42] In addition, with an NPV of 85% on Bethesda category V nodules when the GEC is benign, clinicians may use the GEC information to offer a hemithyroidectomy (with possible completion total thyroidectomy) as opposed to an up-front total thyroidectomy.

Several groups have now reported their clinical experience with the Afirma GEC in routine clinical practice (B Michael, personal communication to RT Kloos, 2013).[10,11,43–47] In the 2 largest series, the GEC result was benign just over half the time, and in this case, patients were managed with observation in lieu of operation 92% to 94% of the time.[10,11] Defining the number needed to test (NNT) as the number of tests needed to be performed to change the clinical outcome of one patient (NNT = 1/[%GEC benign]), then the NNT of these series is 2. Thus, one patient avoids surgery for every 2 patients tested.

Most GEC benign patients in the clinical series reported to date did not undergo surgery, consistent with the purpose of the test (B Michael, personal communication to RT Kloos, 2013).[10,11,43–47] Attempts to validate the GEC test performance on a small set of patients will necessarily result in very wide confidence intervals that are therefore uninterpretable. However, performance can be evaluated among these 654 GEC-tested patients by pooling them together and considering as malignant (false negatives) those GEC benign patients with malignancy found at surgery (4 patients), and as benign (true negatives) those GEC benign patients that underwent surgery and were histologically benign, or were GEC benign and not operated (305 patients). Among these GEC-tested patients across multiple clinical practices, the pooled accuracy of a GEC benign result (NPV) was 99% (95% confidence interval [CI] 96%–100%) (**Fig. 4**) (B Michael, personal communication to RT Kloos, 2013).[11,43–47] Furthermore,

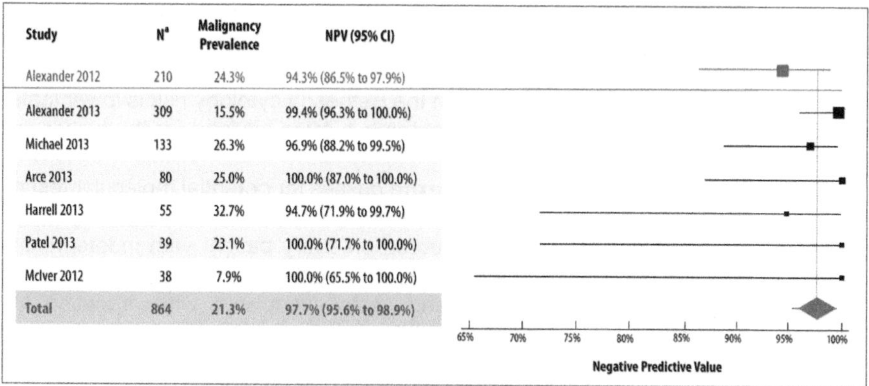

Study	N[a]	Malignancy Prevalence	NPV (95% CI)
Alexander 2012	210	24.3%	94.3% (86.5% to 97.9%)
Alexander 2013	309	15.5%	99.4% (96.3% to 100.0%)
Michael 2013	133	26.3%	96.9% (88.2% to 99.5%)
Arce 2013	80	25.0%	100.0% (87.0% to 100.0%)
Harrell 2013	55	32.7%	94.7% (71.9% to 99.7%)
Patel 2013	39	23.1%	100.0% (71.7% to 100.0%)
McIver 2012	38	7.9%	100.0% (65.5% to 100.0%)
Total	864	21.3%	97.7% (95.6% to 98.9%)

Fig. 4. Consistent Afirma GEC results in real-world clinical experiences recapitulate the clinical validation experience.[7] Outside of the clinical validation experience, the NPV calculation here defines false negatives as GEC benign and histologically malignant, and true negative as GEC benign and histologically benign or unoperated. Statistical calculation method per Newcombe.[74,75] [a] Data include Bethesda III and IV. (*Data from* Refs.[7,11,43–47]; B Michael, personal communication to RT Kloos, 2013.)

the prevalence of malignancy in the GEC suspicious patients (PPV) was 37% (95% CI 32%–43%). Only an adequately trained classifier would demonstrate such reproducible results across 2 prospective independent validation studies[7,8] and these multiple retrospective analyses of clinical experiences that span both academic-based and community-based practices. Given these consistent results, performance remains high after pooling these clinical practice experiences with the Alexander and colleagues[7] prospective clinical validation trial to evaluate the combined experience across these 864 patients (NPV 98% [95% CI 96%–99%], PPV 37% [95% CI 33%–42%]) (see **Fig. 4**). These data demonstrate a very low prevalence of malignancy (1 − NPV) in patients with cytologically indeterminate thyroid nodules that are Afirma GEC benign and support clinical observation in lieu of diagnostic surgery for most GEC benign patients. Of note, without surgical "truth," a limitation of ascertaining true negative status is the variable length of nodule follow-up in the clinical practice studies reported in this pooled analysis. Thus, the meta-analytic NPV may be lower than 98% and clinical observation along with periodic ultrasound (US) assessment of unoperated GEC benign nodules is warranted. Such clinical observation is warranted as well for unoperated cytologically benign nodules given their residual ROM.[38] However, Lee and colleagues[48] found no improved detection of malignancies among cytologically benign nodules when followed longer than 3 years and suggested that stopping routine follow-up after this duration of time should be considered. This consideration may also apply to cytologically indeterminate nodules that are GEC benign. Last, because NPV is impacted by the prevalence of malignancy, and the ROM in the pooled analysis was only 21.3%, the authors calculated the NPV for a higher ROM of 25%. This meta-analytic NPV for the pooled analysis adjusted to 25% ROM remained high at 97% (95% CI 95%–99%).

For the surgeon, in addition to the risk factors of the individual patient, these data inform their clinical decisions for both GEC benign and suspicious patients. For GEC suspicious patients, the ultimate decision is typically between a hemithyroidectomy and a total thyroidectomy. This decision takes into account multiple factors, including imaging findings in the contralateral lobe, the potential value to spare the contralateral thyroid lobe, and the patient's preferences regarding the possible need for a completion thyroidectomy should malignancy be found after hemithyroidectomy. Given the higher risks of laryngeal nerve injury and hypoparathyroidism with a total thyroidectomy versus hemithyroidectomy, and the PPV of the GEC suspicious result, hemithyroidectomy is often preferred when the Bethesda cytology risk is lower (categories III and IV). In contrast, total thyroidectomy is often advised for the higher-risk Bethesda category V.

Optimally, physicians routinely collect 2 extra passes for potential molecular testing with the Afirma GEC on every FNAB they perform, or have on-site rapid cytologic assessment so that the GEC can be collected on every patient with indeterminate cytology during one patient visit (see **Fig. 2**). This patient-centric approach avoids the inconvenience, delayed diagnosis, and costs associated with repeating the FNAB when the first FNAB comes back indeterminate. In addition, it is well known that cytologically indeterminate nodules may not be categorized as indeterminate if they undergo a repeat FNAB.[49] At first glance, a repeat FNAB might seem like a good idea to potentially restratify cytologically indeterminate patients as either cytologically benign or malignant. Unfortunately, this creates a clinical problem for patients whose repeat FNAB is cytologically benign, because their ROM may not be fully reduced to the same risk as if their first FNAB had been cytologically benign.[49,50] The conundrum is accentuated by the fact that the GEC is not indicated for cytologically benign material because this is not cost-effective due to the low PPV that results from the low prevalence of malignancy in this setting, and because the GEC specificity of 70% for cytologically benign nodules will predictably result in a false positive GEC suspicious call in too many cytology-benign nodules.[7] For these reasons, it is recommended that the GEC specimen be collected at the same time as the cytology sample during the first thyroid FNAB. When GEC testing is desired in a patient for whom only cytology was previously collected, the cytology must be repeated along with the GEC collection.

DIAGNOSTIC APPLICATION

Clinical Decision-Making

Analysis of NPV and PPV is important, but what does this mean to the patient in front of the clinician? First, it is important to recognize that their ROM in a cytologically indeterminate nodule, and the resulting NPV of any test, is based on that patient's individual features (eg, their gender, history of childhood radiation treatment, US findings) and the interpreting cytologist's thresholds to use cytology indeterminate categories. The point here is that the prevalence of malignancy seen in the entire practice due to referral patterns does not influence the ROM of the patient at hand. The pretest probability of cancer in each individual patient must be considered before interpreting any test result, genomic or otherwise.

How does one know the ROM established by a cytologist's thresholds to categorize thyroid nodule specimens according to the Bethesda system? The most accurate method would be to operate on all of the patients to establish histologic truth for correlation. In practice, this does not (and should not) happen. A common alternative approach is to combine the results of surgical histology in operated patients with clinical follow-up findings in unoperated patients, making the assumption that unoperated nodules that remain stable in size (with or without stable US characteristics) are histologically benign. A limitation of this approach is that some thyroid cancers can remain stable or grow slowly over years, which falsely lowers the prevalence of malignancy in these series. As a result, follow-up thyroid nodule evaluation has been recommended for at least ~3 years.[48,51] A problem with each of these experimental models is that the results reflect past (and potentially outdated) decisions and thresholds. Veracyte collaborates with Thyroid Cytopathology Partners (TCP) to perform cytology for community-based physicians. This collaboration offers the clinician and patient the benefits of centralized, high-volume,[52] thyroid-only cytopathologists, assures the use of recommended Bethesda diagnostic nomenclature, and offers the opportunity to monitor the rate of utilization of Bethesda indeterminate categories.

One way to approximate the ROM in a particular clinical setting in the absence of surgical histology is to assume that the overall percentage of consecutive cytology indeterminate calls by TCP that are found to be GEC benign (of the total GEC benign plus GEC suspicious samples) is a surrogate for estimating the percentage of truly benign samples, assuming that sensitivity and specificity are as previously reported by Alexander and colleagues.[7] Once ROM is estimated in this manner, one can adjust the NPV of Afirma in these patients using the new prevalence estimate, according to accepted methods. In the first 3617 consecutive GEC calls from TCP read Bethesda III or IV samples in 2013, the percentage of GEC benign was 42%, translating to an estimated 23% ROM and 95% NPV. These data demonstrate that TCP emulates the findings of Alexander and colleagues.[7] These estimates, however, are more accurate in studies with large population numbers that substantially narrow the confidence intervals around the percentage of GEC benign calls in the entire group. In contrast, trying to apply these mathematic models to smaller patient numbers from individual clinical practices leads to uninformatively wide confidence intervals and may produce highly misleading result point estimates of NPV if confidence intervals are not included.

False Negative Results Are the Most Important Diagnostic Error

It is true that as the ROM in a population increases, the NPV declines. However, seeing the NPV decline toward zero as ROM approaches 100% may not give a balanced representation of the risk a false negative Afirma result in clinical practice (**Fig. 5**). True positive and true negative results are correct, and false positive results likely result in surgery in patients who were otherwise destined for surgery by their indeterminate cytology result, so this test error is not a crucial mistake. The main error of concern is a false negative result (eg, a malignant nodule is called GEC benign). Thus, it is important to recognize that the rate of false negative results is capped at 1 − test sensitivity and that given Afirma's 90.2% sensitivity, the risk of false negative calls is limited to a maximum of 9.8% of all test results even when all tested samples are malignant (ROM is 100%) (see **Fig. 5**). More realistic false negative percentages are seen in the Alexander and colleagues study,[7] whereby false negative results (ROM × [1 − sensitivity]) are 2.3%, 2.5%, and 3.6% of all results in Bethesda III, IV, and V specimens, respectively (see **Table 1**). At the individual patient level, the nodule is either malignant or not, so for them all tests perform at either ROM 0% or ROM 100%. For those patients with benign lesions, all GEC benign results are correct calls. For those patients with cancer, their chance of a false negative result is 9.8%. Because approximately 23% of Bethesda III + IV patients have cancer, the occurrence of a false negative result among all Bethesda III + IV patients is 23% × 9.8% = 2.3%. Conversely, the 7 gene mutation DNA panel has a lower sensitivity of 59% in cytologically indeterminate nodules,[29] so the expected maximal false negative percentage is expected to be much higher (41%) (**Fig. 6**).

Suspicious for Hürthle Cell Neoplasm Cytology

In clinical validation, the GEC called only 4 of 21 FNAB samples from Hürthle adenomas as benign (19%).[7] In contrast, in 261 consecutive cytologic Hürthle cell specimens received by TCP between June 2011 and April 2012, 133 were categorized as

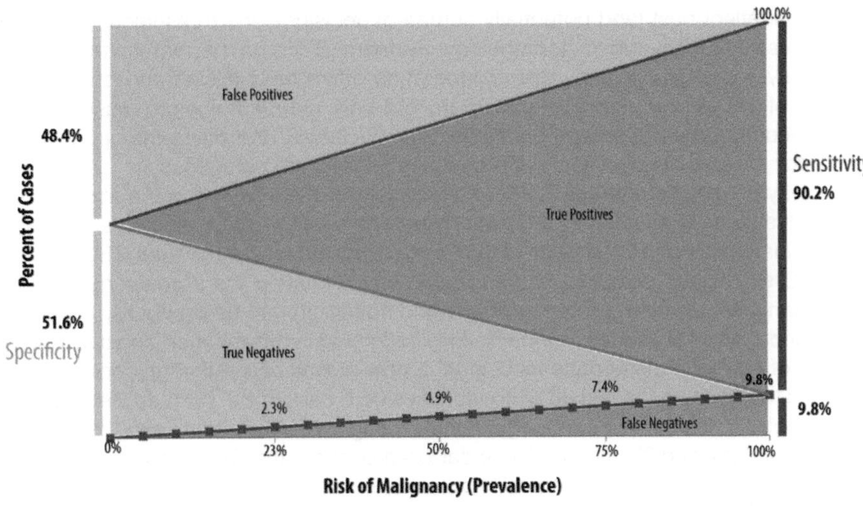

Fig. 5. Afirma GEC false negatives remain low as ROM increases.[7] As ROM increases, true negatives (TN) decrease, and false negatives (FN) increase. Thus, the NPV (NPV = TN/TN + FN) decreases as ROM increases. Although NPV goes to 0% at 100% ROM, false negatives are capped at 1 − sensitivity. Thus, Afirma's high sensitivity limits the occurrence of false negatives. For individual patients, their cytologically indeterminate nodules are either truly benign, or truly malignant, and for them all tests perform at either ROM 0% or ROM 100%.

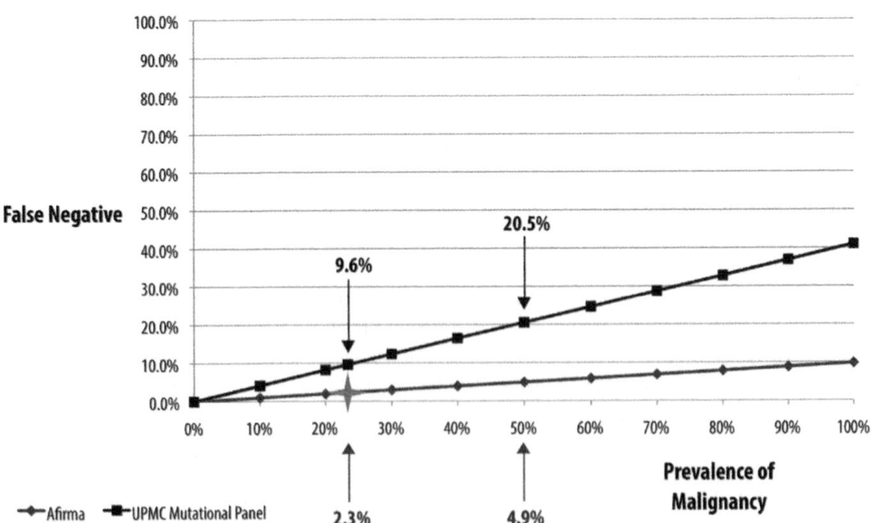

Fig. 6. Occurrence of a false negative result is predicted by ROM × (1 − sensitivity). For individual patients, their cytologically indeterminate nodules are either truly benign, or truly malignant, and for them all tests perform at either ROM 0% or ROM 100%. (*Data from* Alexander EK, Kennedy GC, Baloch ZW, et al. Preoperative diagnosis of benign thyroid nodules with indeterminate cytology. N Engl J Med 2012;367(8):705–15; and Nikiforov YE, Ohori NP, Hodak SP, et al. Impact of mutational testing on the diagnosis and management of patients with cytologically indeterminate thyroid nodules: a prospective analysis of 1056 FNA samples. J Clin Endocrinol Metab 2011;96(11):3390–7.)

Bethesda III and 128 as Bethesda IV. The Afirma GEC called 43% and 42% of these benign, respectively (RT Kloos, unpublished data, 2013). The reason for this apparent discrepancy is that, among cytology samples with Hürthle cell lesions, many are benign histologies that are not Hürthle cell adenomas. Among cytologies suspicious for Hürthle cell neoplasms operated in Alexander and colleagues,[7] most did not end up as Hürthle cell adenomas on postoperative histopathology. In fact, 42% of suspicious for Hürthle cell neoplasm cytology FNABs were found to be benign non-Hürthle adenomas after surgery. Thus, some Hürthle adenomas and many of the non-Hürthle adenomas can potentially be spared unnecessary diagnostic surgery by Afirma with a low risk of a false negative GEC diagnosis. In Alexander and colleagues,[7] there were 2 false negative calls among all Bethesda IV cytologies (2.4%): one cytology was suspicious for a follicular neoplasm, whereas the other was suspicious for a Hürthle cell neoplasm.

However, why does the GEC not call out more Hürthle adenomas as benign? An important reason is that the gold standard histologic diagnosis is highly imperfect. When experts are shown surgical pathology cases, one pathologist identifies the case as a Hürthle carcinoma with either vascular or capsular invasion, whereas 50% to 61% of the time at least one other expert pathologist will call the same lesion benign,[53] causing a problem when training a classifier to recognize "truth." The Afirma GEC and the Hürthle cassette were designed to maximize sensitivity (and therefore NPV and safety) at the expense of specificity (and therefore the PPV and the percentage called benign). As most Hürthle lesions are recommended for surgery, the safely reduced ROM in those cases called GEC benign is the important benefit of the classifier. Specificity is unlikely to be high with any molecular test in Hürthle cell neoplasms given the ambiguity in defining their benign or malignant nature even at surgical pathology.[53] However, as most Hürthle cell lesions are not Hürthle cell neoplasms (Hürthle adenomas or carcinomas), and the GEC calls about 42% of Hürthle cell lesions GEC benign, the test offers the opportunity to safely reduce unnecessary surgery in this broad group of patients as well.

Rare Neoplasms

The Afirma GEC process includes screening filters for MTC, parathyroid tissue, and metastases to the thyroid from renal cell carcinoma, breast carcinoma, and malignant melanoma. Given the rarity of renal cell carcinoma, breast carcinoma, and melanoma metastasis to the thyroid gland, experience is limited and comprehensive clinical validation of these genomic cassettes may take years. However, more extensive experience with the MTC and parathyroid cassettes suggests their validity and utility in planning the extent of and approach to surgery.

The cytologic diagnosis of MTC is challenging.[54] The tumor is uncommon and its cytologic features overlap with those of other neoplasms. When the cytopathologist wrongly suspects MTC, these false positive diagnoses lower cytologic specificity.[55–58] More significant is that nonspecific cytologic features may wrongly suggest tumors other than MTC. These false negative diagnoses result in the failure to cytologically diagnose MTC and lower cytologic sensitivity for MTC.[54,55,57–64] An abstract reporting 14 samples (from 13 patients) that positively expressed the MTC gene expression signature in the Afirma GEC rare neoplasm cassettes found that all 14 were confirmed as MTC on histopathology.[41] Experience with a larger number of MTC cases is needed before stronger conclusions can be drawn about the test's specificity, although high specificity would fill an important clinical gap because the main drawback of serum calcitonin screening for MTC is its high false positive rate.[65] Of the 265 histologically confirmed specimens reported by Alexander and colleagues,[7] none of the 263 non-MTC specimens triggered the MTC cassette, so early findings suggest high specificity. Of the 2 MTCs encountered in the cohort, both were identified by the MTC cassette. In this limited setting, the authors findings suggest that the MTC rare neoplasm cassette has both high PPV and high NPV. A preoperative diagnosis of MTC impacts the patient preoperative evaluation, including evaluation for multiple endocrine neoplasia type 2 (MEN2), and the risk of concomitant pheochromocytoma and hyperparathyroidism. In addition, surgical management is altered to include a minimum of total thyroidectomy and central neck dissection.[66] Finally, preoperative RET proto-oncogene status may alter the management of unintentionally devascularized parathyroid glands among those MEN2 patients at high risk of future hyperparathyroidism.[66] As the preoperative identification of MTC alters clinical management of all patients, the use of an MTC GEC may be appropriate not only for cytologically indeterminate cytology specimens (Bethesda categories III and IV) but also for those that are suspicious for malignancy or malignant (Bethesda V and VI, respectively).

The parathyroid tissue cassette is triggered somewhat less frequently than the MTC cassette, and preliminary findings regarding PPV and NPV are encouraging. Here too clinical management is altered by prompting evaluation for primary or secondary hyperparathyroidism, and, if surgery is indicated, typically altering surgery away from resection of the thyroid to a minimally invasive parathyroid procedure.[67]

Clinical Utility and Cost-Effectiveness

The impact of the Afirma GEC on the physician decision to operate when the FNAB cytology is indeterminate and the Afirma GEC result is benign has been reported in 2 published multicenter studies. Duick and colleagues[10] reported on the initial 2040 consecutive indeterminate thyroid FNAB biopsies collected in clinical practice. Fifty-two percent of these cytologically indeterminate samples were GEC benign. Thus, the NNT for the GEC equals 2. Physicians adopted watchful waiting in lieu of diagnostic thyroid surgery 92.4% of the time when the Afirma GEC result reclassified the cytologically indeterminate nodule as benign. In contrast to the 73% to 74% historical rate of diagnostic surgery on cytologically indeterminate thyroid nodules,[4,53] 7.6% of those that were Afirma GEC benign proceeded to surgery, a dramatic 90% reduction in the decision to operate ($P<.001$).[10] The decision to operate was not statistically different from the 9% operative rate on patients with benign cytology diagnoses reported in a recent meta-review.[4] Physicians who elected surgery for patients with an Afirma GEC benign result reported similar reasons to operate as those found for operated cytologically benign nodules (eg, large nodule, compression, other suspicious nodule, rapid nodule growth).[10]

Similarly, Alexander and colleagues[11] performed an independent multicenter investigation of 339 cytologically indeterminate (Bethesda III–V) nodules aspirated at 5 academic centers. Fifty-one percent of the GEC results were benign, again demonstrating an NNT = 2. In addition, 41% of the cohort had follow-up data (1–24 months). Thyroid surgery occurred in 6.3% of GEC benign patients compared with 81.8% of GEC suspicious patients. Among GEC benign patients, there was 1 false negative patient who had a 1.0-cm nodule on US that proved to be a 6-mm papillary carcinoma when surgically resected (NPV 98.6% when defining “benign” as histologically benign, or GEC benign and not operated). Forty-four percent of GEC suspicious patients who underwent surgery were found to harbor malignancy in the thyroid nodule of interest. The authors concluded that their experience confirmed the performance characteristics of the GEC and its clinical utility.[11]

An independent incremental cost-effectiveness study found no difference in missed cancers between paradigms that did or did not use the Afirma GEC in a Markov model using 10,000 Monte Carlo simulations of the expected range of probabilities for different potential outcomes.[13] However, they did find that the Afirma paradigm reduced direct health care costs by $4953 per 5-year episode of care, allowing $1453 in direct savings using the then current Medicare reimbursement rates for surgery and the Afirma test, while modestly improving quality of life by 0.07 quality-adjusted life-years.[13] This cost-savings estimate was conservative because it projected a 14% rate of operation on GEC benign thyroid nodules (based on expert opinion), a rate that proved to be double the rates subsequently reported in actual clinical practice.[10,11] Re-evaluating the cost-effectiveness of the Afirma GEC assuming that 7.6% of GEC benign patients would undergo surgery, each test would save $2600.[10] These cost savings are substantially eroded when the physician does not collect the GEC with the first FNAB, which requires the patient to return for another US-guided FNAB to collect the GEC and concomitant cytologic specimen. For example, the cost of performing a US-guided FNAB is approximately $650 in the clinic setting and $1100 in the hospital outpatient setting at the Medicare National Payment Amount (www.CMS.gov 2013 Physician Fee Schedule). In addition to adding health care expense, the delay in time to the second FNAB is not optimal for the patient because it prolongs their time of diagnostic uncertainty and delays the time to an actionable result.

Understanding the cost of a test requires an understanding of who is paying for the testing service. There is the list price charged to third-party insurers, the contracted price that an insurer negotiates to pay for the test, and the cost to the patient (including remaining deductibles and copayments). Veracyte accepts all insurance and protects underserved and underinsured patients from high out-of-pocket costs with the Afirma Access patient assistance program. Patients with Medicare fee-for-service insurance are billed a 20% copayment of approximately $30 for cytology per nodule when the sample is sent to TCP. However, Medicare fully covers the cost of the GEC with no out-of-pocket charge because it is reimbursed on the Clinical Lab Fee Schedule, which carries no deductibles or copayments for beneficiaries. Veracyte bills noncontracted third-party insurance carriers the GEC list price. When the claim is unpaid or processed as an out-of-network service with high cost share for the patient, the Afirma Access program dramatically reduces or waives the patient's out-of-pocket responsibility based on their household income. For example, in 2013 a family of 4 earning less than $89,400 pays nothing out of pocket under the Afirma Access program (Veracyte Inc Afirma Access Program 2013). If the patient's third-party insurer is contracted with Veracyte and the GEC claim is processed as an in-network service, the patient is billed their in-network laboratory copayment (typically 10%) and any deductible as they would with any other in-network service. Low-income patients still qualify for the Afirma Access program to reduce or waive their out-of-pocket expenses. If the GEC fails quality control due to insufficient RNA quantity or quality, neither the patient nor the third-party insurer is billed for the test.

Future Directions

Future opportunities exist to identify rare neoplasms among nodules that are cytologically suspicious for malignancy or cytologically malignant. Additional opportunities may include the development of a "rule-in" classifier with high PPV. Such a classifier may be useful to identify malignancy in Afirma GEC suspicious nodules to direct an optimal initial treatment (eg, total thyroidectomy instead of a diagnostic hemithyroidectomy that then requires a second surgery for completion thyroidectomy). To this end, early feasibility indicates it is possible to accurately assign BRAF mutational status by examining gene expression patterns in the same RNA sample on which Afirma GEC testing is currently performed.[68]

Ideally, the decision to operate and the extent of the operation could be determined via one diagnostic FNAB sample through a high-sensitivity/high NPV and high-specificity/high PPV test (or series of tests) with a cost that reduces overall health care costs. Currently no single test offers both of these diagnostic characteristics. The development of such a test through the discovery of relevant biomarkers or GEC classifiers alone, in combination, or in series using current or emerging technologies may further alter the management of patients with thyroid nodules.

SUMMARY

The introduction of thyroid FNAB dramatically reduced unnecessary diagnostic thyroid surgery by rendering an actionable result when the cytologic diagnosis was benign, suspicious for malignancy, or malignant. Among patients with cytologically benign lesions, the ROM is low, and this combined with the generally indolent nature of thyroid cancer has led clinicians to follow these patients conservatively and avoid diagnostic surgery. In the minority of the patients where FNAB cytology is indeterminate, most patients have been referred for diagnostic surgery given the higher ROM.[3] The application of molecular diagnostics to these cytologically indeterminate samples now offers the opportunity to improve patient care by clarifying this diagnostic ambiguity and avoiding surgeries on thyroid nodules unlikely to be malignant (chance of being benign = NPV).

Mutational panels and the Afirma GEC tests do not provide the same information. The Afirma GEC is the only test with high sensitivity (90.2%), with published clinical validation established via a prospective multicenter study involving academic and community practices where the GEC result was compared with the gold standard histopathological truth, which was rendered by a panel of thyroid pathology experts who were "blinded" to the GEC result. When the Afirma GEC is benign, there is a very low chance that the result is falsely negative (ROM × [1 − sensitivity]). At a typical 23% ROM for indeterminate lesions (Bethesda III and IV), the chance of a false negative result is just 2.3%. If one unrealistically doubles this ROM, the chance of a false negative result remains acceptably low at 4.5%. Thus, combined with good clinical judgment for the individual patient, most GEC benign patients can safely avoid diagnostic surgery. Sensitivity and specificity have been published for some, but not all, point mutation/gene rearrangement panels (with or without microRNA analysis) in cytologically indeterminate nodules (see **Fig. 1**). At this time, the Afirma GEC is the only molecular test that has published clinical utility studies showing that observation is substituted for surgery in either academic-based or community-based practices when the GEC result is benign. In contrast, DNA point mutations or rearrangements lack sensitivity in Bethesda III/IV nodules; thus, when these alterations are not found (which occurs in approximately 40% of the malignancies), cancer cannot be confidently excluded, so surgery is still indicated. High sensitivity is critical to rule out cancer, because the test must identify most cancerous nodules to reliably identify nodules that are benign. The Afirma GEC mRNA Classifier has the highest test sensitivity among all available approaches to preoperatively address cytologically indeterminate nodules and is recommended in cases where lowering unnecessary surgery is desired.

REFERENCES

1. Cooper DS, Doherty GM, Haugen BR, et al. Revised American Thyroid Association management guidelines for patients with thyroid nodules and differentiated thyroid cancer. Thyroid 2009;19(11):1167–214.

2. Hegedus L. Clinical practice. The thyroid nodule. N Engl J Med 2004;351(17): 1764–71.
3. Melillo RM, Santoro M. Molecular biomarkers in thyroid FNA samples. J Clin Endocrinol Metab 2012;97(12):4370–3.
4. Wang CC, Friedman L, Kennedy GC, et al. A large multicenter correlation study of thyroid nodule cytopathology and histopathology. Thyroid 2011;21(3): 243–51.
5. Bryson PC, Shores CG, Hart C, et al. Immunohistochemical distinction of follicular thyroid adenomas and follicular carcinomas. Arch Otolaryngol Head Neck Surg 2008;134(6):581–6.
6. Xing M, Haugen BR, Schlumberger M. Progress in molecular-based management of differentiated thyroid cancer. Lancet 2013;381(9871):1058–69.
7. Alexander EK, Kennedy GC, Baloch ZW, et al. Preoperative diagnosis of benign thyroid nodules with indeterminate cytology. N Engl J Med 2012;367(8):705–15.
8. Chudova D, Wilde JI, Wang ET, et al. Molecular classification of thyroid nodules using high-dimensionality genomic data. J Clin Endocrinol Metab 2010;95(12): 5296–304.
9. Walsh PS, Wilde JI, Tom EY, et al. Analytical performance verification of a molecular diagnostic for cytology-indeterminate thyroid nodules. J Clin Endocrinol Metab 2012;97(12):E2297–306.
10. Duick DS, Klopper JP, Diggans JC, et al. The impact of benign gene expression classifier test results on the endocrinologist-patient decision to operate on patients with thyroid nodules with indeterminate fine-needle aspiration cytopathology. Thyroid 2012;22(10):996–1001.
11. Alexander EK, Schorr M, Klopper J, et al. Multicenter clinical experience with the afirma gene expression classifier. J Clin Endocrinol Metab 2014;99(1):119–25.
12. Parker CA, Steward DL. Impact of the gene expression classifier on surgeon-patient decision making in indeterminate thyroid nodules [abstract]. Otolaryngol Head Neck Surg 2013;149(No. 2 Suppl):P49.
13. Li H, Robinson KA, Anton B, et al. Cost-effectiveness of a novel molecular test for cytologically indeterminate thyroid nodules. J Clin Endocrinol Metab 2011; 96(11):E1719–26.
14. Saravanan P, Chau WF, Roberts N, et al. Psychological well-being in patients on 'adequate' doses of l-thyroxine: results of a large, controlled community-based questionnaire study. Clin Endocrinol 2002;57(5):577–85.
15. Cooper DS, Biondi B. Subclinical thyroid disease. Lancet 2012;379(9821): 1142–54.
16. Shrime MG, Goldstein DP, Seaberg RM, et al. Cost-effective management of low-risk papillary thyroid carcinoma. Arch Otolaryngol Head Neck Surg 2007; 133(12):1245–53.
17. Esnaola NF, Cantor SB, Sherman SI, et al. Optimal treatment strategy in patients with papillary thyroid cancer: a decision analysis. Surgery 2001;130(6): 921–30.
18. Hundahl SA, Cady B, Cunningham MP, et al. Initial results from a prospective cohort study of 5583 cases of thyroid carcinoma treated in the United States during 1996. U.S. and German Thyroid Cancer Study Group. An American College of Surgeons Commission on Cancer Patient Care Evaluation study. Cancer 2000;89(1):202–17.
19. Bergenfelz A, Jansson S, Kristoffersson A, et al. Complications to thyroid surgery: results as reported in a database from a multicenter audit comprising 3,660 patients. Langenbecks Arch Surg 2008;393(5):667–73.

20. Chandrasekhar SS, Randolph GW, Seidman MD, et al. Clinical practice guideline: improving voice outcomes after thyroid surgery. Otolaryngol Head Neck Surg 2013;148(Suppl 6):S1–37.
21. Young WG, Succar E, Hsu L, et al. Causes of emergency department visits following thyroid and parathyroid surgery. JAMA Otolaryngol Head Neck Surg 2013;139(11):1175–80.
22. Sosa JA, Bowman HM, Tielsch JM, et al. The importance of surgeon experience for clinical and economic outcomes from thyroidectomy. Ann Surg 1998;228(3):320–30.
23. Saunders BD, Wainess RM, Dimick JB, et al. Who performs endocrine operations in the United States? Surgery 2003;134(6):924–31 [discussion: 931].
24. Veenstra DL, Piper M, Haddow JE, et al. Improving the efficiency and relevance of evidence-based recommendations in the era of whole-genome sequencing: an EGAPP methods update. Genet Med 2013;15(1):14–24.
25. Teutsch SM, Bradley LA, Palomaki GE, et al. The Evaluation of Genomic Applications in Practice and Prevention (EGAPP) Initiative: methods of the EGAPP Working Group. Genet Med 2009;11(1):3–14.
26. Tuckson RV, Newcomer L, De Sa JM. Accessing genomic medicine: affordability, diffusion, and disparities. JAMA 2013;309(14):1469–70.
27. Ali SZ, Fish SA, Lanman R, et al. Use of the afirma(R) gene expression classifier for preoperative identification of benign thyroid nodules with indeterminate fine needle aspiration cytopathology. PLoS Curr 2013;5. pii: ecurrents.eogt.e557cbb5c7e4f66568ce582a373057e7.
28. Grody WW, Thompson BH, Hudgins L. Whole-exome/genome sequencing and genomics. Pediatrics 2013;132(Suppl 3):S211–5.
29. Nikiforov YE, Ohori NP, Hodak SP, et al. Impact of mutational testing on the diagnosis and management of patients with cytologically indeterminate thyroid nodules: a prospective analysis of 1056 FNA samples. J Clin Endocrinol Metab 2011;96(11):3390–7.
30. Keutgen XM, Filicori F, Crowley MJ, et al. A panel of four miRNAs accurately differentiates malignant from benign indeterminate thyroid lesions on fine needle aspiration. Clin Cancer Res 2012;18(7):2032–8.
31. Jameson JL. Minimizing unnecessary surgery for thyroid nodules. N Engl J Med 2012;367(8):765–7.
32. NCCN Clinical Practice Guidelines in Oncology. Thyroid Carcinoma. NCCN Clinical Practice Guidelines in Oncology 2013; Version 1.2013. Available at: http://www.nccn.org/professionals/physician_gls/pdf/thyroid.pdf. Accessed January 9, 2013.
33. Ferraz C, Eszlinger M, Paschke R. Current state and future perspective of molecular diagnosis of fine-needle aspiration biopsy of thyroid nodules. J Clin Endocrinol Metab 2011;96(7):2016–26.
34. Wiseman SM, Haddad Z, Walker B, et al. Whole-transcriptome profiling of thyroid nodules identifies expression-based signatures for accurate thyroid cancer diagnosis. J Clin Endocrinol Metab 2013;98(10):4072–9.
35. Shrestha M, Crothers BA, Burch HB. The impact of thyroid nodule size on the risk of malignancy and accuracy of fine-needle aspiration: a 10-year study from a single institution. Thyroid 2012;22(12):1251–6.
36. Lewis CM, Chang KP, Pitman M, et al. Thyroid fine-needle aspiration biopsy: variability in reporting. Thyroid 2009;19(7):717–23.
37. Borget I, Vielh P, Leboulleux S, et al. Assessment of the cost of fine-needle aspiration cytology as a diagnostic tool in patients with thyroid nodules. Am J Clin Pathol 2008;129(5):763–71.

38. Renshaw A. An estimate of risk of malignancy for a benign diagnosis in thyroid fine-needle aspirates. Cancer Cytopathol 2010;118(4):190–5.
39. Marchevsky AM, Walts AE, Bose S, et al. Evidence-based evaluation of the risks of malignancy predicted by thyroid fine-needle aspiration biopsies. Diagn Cytopathol 2010;38(4):252–9.
40. Spitalnic S. Test properties 2: likelihood ratios, Bayes' formula, and receiver operating curves. Hosp Physician 2004;40(10):53–8.
41. Kloos RT, O'Reilly K, Traweek ST, et al. Novel Gene Expression Classifier Raises Pre-Operative Suspicion of Medullary Thyroid Cancer [abstract]. Paper presented at: AACE 21st Annual Scientific and Clinical Congress. Philadelphia, May 23–27, 2012.
42. Monroe R, Vora A, Kloos RT, et al. Novel gene expression classifier raises preoperative suspicion of medullary thyroid carcinoma in FNAs with hürthle cell neoplasm cytology [abstract]. Journal of the American Society of Cytopathology 2013;2(Suppl 1):S82.
43. Arce KM, Mohan V, Desantis P, et al. Clinical validity and utility of the novel gene expression classifier in thyroid nodules at Cleveland Clinic Florida [abstract]. Thyroid 2013;23(S1):A54–5.
44. Harrell RM, Bimston DN. Surgical utility of afirma: effects of high cancer prevalence and oncocytic cell types in patients with indeterminate thyroid cytology. Endocr Pract 2013;20(4):364–9.
45. Patel KN, Heller KS. The benefit of gene expression classifier testing in avoiding surgery on indeterminate thyroid nodules may be less than anticipated [abstract]. Thyroid 2013;23(S1):A40.
46. Michael B, Harrell RM, Hands K. A Community-based evaluation of the Afirma gene expression classifier (GEC) in indeterminate thyroid nodules [abstract]. American Association of Clinical Endocrinologists Annual Meeting. Phoenix, May, 2013. p. 186.
47. McIver B, Reddi HV, Kosok LL, et al. An independent study of a gene expression classifier (Afirma) in the evaluation of cytologically indeterminate thyroid nodules: initial report [abstract]. Thyroid 2012;22(S1):A81–2.
48. Lee S, Skelton TS, Zheng F, et al. The biopsy-proven benign thyroid nodule: is long-term follow-up necessary? J Am Coll Surg 2013;217(1):81–8 [discussion: 88–9].
49. VanderLaan PA, Marqusee E, Krane JF. Clinical outcome for atypia of undetermined significance in thyroid fine-needle aspirations: should repeated FNA be the preferred initial approach? Am J Clin Pathol 2011;135(5):770–5.
50. Renshaw AA. Does a repeated benign aspirate change the risk of malignancy after an initial atypical thyroid fine-needle aspiration? Am J Clin Pathol 2010;134(5):788–92.
51. Nou E, Kwong N, Alexander LK, et al. Determination of the optimal time interval for repeat evaluation following a benign thyroid nodule aspiration. J Clin Endocrinol Metab 2014;99(2):510–6.
52. Halm EA, Lee C, Chassin MR. Is volume related to outcome in health care? A systematic review and methodologic critique of the literature. Ann Intern Med 2002;137(6):511–20.
53. Cibas ES, Baloch ZW, Fellegara G, et al. A prospective assessment defining the limitations of thyroid nodule pathologic evaluation. Ann Intern Med 2013;159(5):325–32.
54. Essig GF, Porter K, Schneider D, et al. Fine needle aspiration and medullary thyroid carcinoma: the risk of inadequate preoperative evaluation and initial surgery when relying upon FNAB cytology alone. Endocr Pract 2013;19(6):920–7.

55. Lew JI, Snyder RA, Sanchez YM, et al. Fine needle aspiration of the thyroid: correlation with final histopathology in a surgical series of 797 patients. J Am Coll Surg 2011;213(1):188–94 [discussion: 194–5].
56. Papaparaskeva K, Nagel H, Droese M. Cytologic diagnosis of medullary carcinoma of the thyroid gland. Diagn Cytopathol 2000;22(6):351–8.
57. Shah SS, Faquin WC, Izquierdo R, et al. FNA of misclassified primary malignant neoplasms of the thyroid: impact on clinical management. Cytojournal 2009;6:1.
58. Jo VY, Stelow EB, Dustin SM, et al. Malignancy risk for fine-needle aspiration of thyroid lesions according to the Bethesda System for Reporting Thyroid Cytopathology. Am J Clin Pathol 2010;134(3):450–6.
59. Choi N, Moon WJ, Lee JH, et al. Ultrasonographic findings of medullary thyroid cancer: differences according to tumor size and correlation with fine needle aspiration results. Acta Radiol 2011;52(3):312–6.
60. Bugalho MJ, Santos JR, Sobrinho L. Preoperative diagnosis of medullary thyroid carcinoma: fine needle aspiration cytology as compared with serum calcitonin measurement. J Surg Oncol 2005;91(1):56–60.
61. Kudo T, Miyauchi A, Ito Y, et al. Diagnosis of medullary thyroid carcinoma by calcitonin measurement in fine-needle aspiration biopsy specimens. Thyroid 2007;17(7):635–8.
62. Dustin SM, Jo VY, Hanley KZ, et al. High sensitivity and positive predictive value of fine-needle aspiration for uncommon thyroid malignancies. Diagn Cytopathol 2012;40(5):416–21.
63. Elisei R, Bottici V, Luchetti F, et al. Impact of routine measurement of serum calcitonin on the diagnosis and outcome of medullary thyroid cancer: experience in 10,864 patients with nodular thyroid disorders. J Clin Endocrinol Metab 2004; 89(1):163–8.
64. Fischer AH, Clayton AC, Bentz JS, et al. Performance differences between conventional smears and liquid-based preparations of thyroid fine-needle aspiration samples: analysis of 47,076 responses in the College of American Pathologists Interlaboratory Comparison Program in Non-Gynecologic Cytology. Arch Pathol Lab Med 2013;137(1):26–31.
65. Costante G, Durante C, Francis Z, et al. Determination of calcitonin levels in C-cell disease: clinical interest and potential pitfalls. Nat Clin Pract Endocrinol Metab 2009;5(1):35–44.
66. Kloos RT, Eng C, Evans DB, et al. Medullary thyroid cancer: management guidelines of the American Thyroid Association. Thyroid 2009;19(6):565–612.
67. Bischoff LA, Curry J, Jabbour S, et al. Pitfalls in indeterminate cytopathology of "thyroid" nodules [abstract]. Thyroid 2013;23(S1):A104.
68. Kennedy GC, diggans J, Walsh S, et al. Classification of BRAF V600E status using high-dimensional RNA expression data [abstract]. Thyroid 2013;23(S1):A39.
69. Nikiforova MN, Wald AI, Roy S, et al. Targeted next-generation sequencing panel (ThyroSeq) for detection of mutations in thyroid cancer. J Clin Endocrinol Metab 2013;98(11):E1852–60.
70. Gharib H, Papini E, Paschke R, et al. American Association of Clinical Endocrinologists, Associazione Medici Endocrinologi, and European Thyroid Association Medical guidelines for clinical practice for the diagnosis and management of thyroid nodules: executive summary of recommendations. Endocr Pract 2010;16(3): 468–75.
71. Yassa L, Cibas ES, Benson CB, et al. Long-term assessment of a multidisciplinary approach to thyroid nodule diagnostic evaluation. Cancer 2007;111(6): 508–16.

72. Haugen BR, Baloch Ż, Chudova D, et al. Development of a novel molecular classifier to accurately identify benign thyroid nodules in patients with indeterminate FNA cytology [abstract]. 14th International Thyroid Congress. Paris (France), September, 2010.
73. Cibas ES, Ali SZ. The Bethesda system for reporting thyroid cytopathology. Thyroid 2009;19(11):1159–65.
74. Newcombe RG. Two-sided confidence intervals for the single proportion: comparison of seven methods. Stat Med 1998;17(8):857–72.
75. Lowry R. VassarStats: Website for Statistical Computation. Available at: http://vassarstats.net/index.html. Accessed December 1, 2013.

The Prognostic Implications from Molecular Testing of Thyroid Cancer

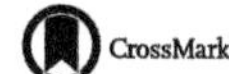

Ozan B. Ozgursoy, MD[a], David W. Eisele, MD[a], Ralph P. Tufano, MD, MBA[b,*]

KEYWORDS

- Thyroid cancer • Prognosis • Molecular genetics • BRAF • RAS • RET/PTC • PAX8-PPAR • Targeted therapy

KEY POINTS

- Molecular testing offers valuable information for the management and prognosis of patients with thyroid cancer by detecting genetic alterations.
- Molecular markers may guide clinicians to assess the individual risk of recurrence and metastasis from thyroid cancer and to tailor the treatment according to that risk stratification.
- B-type RAF mutation has emerged as a possible marker for more aggressive behavior of papillary thyroid cancer; RET/PTC may be a marker of more favorable thyroid tumor behavior.
- There are currently no prospective, well-defined data supporting the use of molecular markers alone to decide on the extent of treatment or to predict the prognosis in patients with thyroid cancer.
- Molecular markers are promising targets for novel therapies and, in particular, for thyroid cancers with aggressive behavior.

INTRODUCTION

Thyroid cancer is the most common endocrine malignancy and accounts for approximately 1% of all newly diagnosed cancers. A significant worldwide increase in the incidence of thyroid cancer has been noted over the past few decades.

Disclosures: None.

[a] Department of Otolaryngology-Head and Neck Surgery, Johns Hopkins Outpatient Center, The Johns Hopkins University School of Medicine, 601 North Caroline Street, 6th Floor, Baltimore, MD 21287, USA; [b] Division of Head and Neck Endocrine Surgery, Department of Otolaryngology-Head and Neck Surgery, Johns Hopkins Outpatient Center, The Johns Hopkins University School of Medicine, 601 North Caroline Street, 6th Floor, Baltimore, MD 21287, USA
* Corresponding author.
E-mail address: rtufano1@jhmi.edu

Otolaryngol Clin N Am 47 (2014) 595–607
http://dx.doi.org/10.1016/j.otc.2014.04.010
oto.theclinics.com
0030-6665/14/$ – see front matter

Age-standardized incidence of thyroid cancer in developed countries is estimated to be 9.1 per 100,000 women and 2.9 per 100,000 men.[1] Papillary thyroid carcinoma is almost entirely responsible for the overall increase in the incidence of thyroid cancer in the last several decades. There is also an increase in the incidence of diagnosed thyroid nodules that parallels the rapid increase in the incidence of thyroid cancer. The prevalence of thyroid nodules on physical examination is almost 10% in adults and is detected at a higher rate (up to 70%) in the elderly population if thyroid ultrasonography is used. It is crucial to distinguish cancer from benign thyroid nodules because there is an overall 5% to 10% risk of malignancy in thyroid nodules.[2]

Most of the thyroid cancers are epithelial, follicular cell derived, and the most frequent type is papillary thyroid carcinoma, which constitutes more than 80% of all thyroid malignancies. The second most frequent type of thyroid cancer is follicular thyroid carcinoma, which accounts for 10% to 15% of all thyroid malignancies.[1–4] Follicular carcinoma most likely originates either from a preexisting benign follicular adenoma or directly, bypassing the stage of adenoma.[2,3] Medullary thyroid carcinomas, which account for approximately 3% of all thyroid malignancies, develop from the parafollicular C cells of the thyroid gland. Anaplastic and poorly differentiated thyroid carcinomas are rare but represent the most aggressive types, with high mortality.[1] Papillary and follicular thyroid carcinomas, the so-called differentiated thyroid cancers, constitute more than 90% of all thyroid malignancies and they are usually associated with a good prognosis because most have an indolent course. The classic treatment of choice for thyroid cancer is total thyroidectomy with or without radioactive iodine. Despite high disease recurrence rates of up to 20% to 30% in differentiated thyroid cancers, the overall prognosis is still favorable, with a 10-year survival rate of more than 90%. However, surgically inoperable or radioiodine-resistant differentiated thyroid cancers do not yet have an effective treatment and can still cause death.[1–4]

The prognostic factors favoring recurrence, metastasis, and death from differentiated thyroid cancer include both patient and tumor factors. Among patient factors are age less than 15 years or more than 45 years, male sex, and family history of thyroid cancer.[4] Tumor factors include a primary tumor larger than 2 cm, multifocal cancer, nuclear atypia, tumor necrosis, vascular invasion, extrathyroidal extension, lymph node metastasis, distant metastasis, tall cell and columnar cell variants, and radioiodine resistance.[4] A poor prognosis is most commonly associated with neck recurrence caused by lymph node metastasis or thyroid bed remnant disease and less commonly with distant metastasis.[4]

It can be challenging to assess the individual risk for recurrence and metastasis of thyroid cancer and tailor the treatment according to that risk stratification. However, recent investigations have made progress in understanding the molecular mechanisms of thyroid cancer. These investigations have revealed that thyroid cancers frequently have genetic alterations, and current molecular studies can detect these alterations and offer valuable information for diagnosis, management, and prognosis of patients with thyroid cancer. This article discusses the current use of molecular markers for thyroid cancer from a prognostic and therapeutic perspective.

RELEVANT PATHOPHYSIOLOGY

Genetic Alteration of Mitogen-activated Protein Kinase Signaling Pathway

The mitogen-activated protein kinase (MAPK) signaling pathway is an intracellular cascade regulating division, proliferation, differentiation, adhesion, migration, and apoptosis in the cell. This pathway also plays a role in survival in response to growth factors, hormones, and cytokines that interact with cell surface receptor tyrosine kinases.[2,5] Aberrant activation of MAPK pathway has been described in some human malignancies, including thyroid cancer.[2,5,6] B-type RAF (BRAF) mutation, RET/PTC rearrangement, and RAS mutation are the common triggers for the activation of the MAPK signaling pathway. When this pathway is activated in the thyroid cells by various growth factors and hormones, a G protein–coupled receptor on the plasma membrane can be activated. This activated G protein RAS then activates the serine/threonine protein kinase RAF. The activation of this cascade has a role in thyroid tumorigenesis by altering some of the cellular functions, which are discussed later.[2,5]

BRAF Mutation

BRAF is the predominant isoform of the RAF proteins in follicular thyroid cells and is a potent activator of the MAPK signaling pathway. BRAF-induced activation of the MAPK pathway interferes with cellular communication, division, differentiation, proliferation, and apoptosis, and therefore plays a role in several disease processes, such as chronic inflammation and cancer.[5,6]

BRAF mutation involves nucleotide 1799 and results in a valine-to-glutamate substitution at residue 600 (V600E) of the BRAF protein, and this is the most common genetic alteration in papillary thyroid carcinoma. BRAF mutation is highly prevalent in classic papillary carcinoma and the tall cell variant, whereas it is rare in the follicular variant.[1–5] The other rare mutation of the BRAF gene results in a lysine-to-glutamate substitution at residue 601 of the BRAF protein. This BRAF (K601E) mutation has been found particularly in the follicular variant of papillary thyroid carcinoma. This article uses BRAF mutation to denote the BRAF(V600E) mutation. Moreover, a chromosomal rearrangement, the AKAP/BRAF rearrangement, has been suggested to be associated with papillary thyroid carcinoma in patients exposed to radiation.[2,5]

RET/PTC Rearrangement

The RET proto-oncogene is structurally related to tyrosine kinase transmembrane receptors and is involved in glial cell–derived neurotropic factor signaling.[5] RET/PTC rearrangement is a result of a fusion between the 3′ portion of the RET receptor tyrosine kinase gene and the 5′ portion of an unrelated gene.[2] RET/PTC rearrangement can activate the MAPK pathway but the oncogenic effects of this rearrangement in thyroid tumorigenesis require signaling along that pathway in the presence of functional BRAF kinase.[7]

RET/PTC rearrangement has been found to be more common in post-Chernobyl thyroid cancers, and is therefore suggested to be associated with radiation exposure. However, it has also been found in adenomas as well as the other benign tumors of the thyroid gland.[2]

RAS Mutation

The RAS family contains more than 50 small proteins that relay signals from tyrosine kinase receptors and G protein–coupled receptors. RAS is linked to the inner cell membrane and plays a role in the intracellular transduction of signals arising from cell membrane receptors.[2,5] In its active state, RAS protein activates the MAPK and some other signaling pathways. Mutations in the RAS gene result in formation of a mutant protein that potentially has an oncogenic effect in the development of thyroid cancer.[2] It has been reported that point mutations result in constitutive activation of the RAS protein and lead to the induction of a malignant phenotype, with cell proliferation, invasion, metastasis, and resistance to apoptosis in some human cancers, including thyroid cancer.[8]

PAX8-PPAR Rearrangement

PAX8-PPAR rearrangement results from a translocation that leads to fusion of PAX8 and PPAR genes.[2,5] PAX8 is a transcription factor regulating the expression of some thyroid-specific genes and proliferation/differentiation of thyroid follicular cells. PPAR is also a transcription factor that is a member of a hormone nuclear receptor family, and it is slightly expressed in normal thyroid tissue.[5] PAX8-PPAR rearrangement has been encountered in follicular thyroid carcinoma and the follicular variant of papillary thyroid carcinoma, and rarely in Hürthle cell thyroid carcinoma. However, the role of this rearrangement in the development of thyroid cancers is not yet clearly understood.[5]

CLINICAL PRESENTATION AND EXAMINATION

Cytologic assessment by fine-needle aspiration biopsy (FNAB) has been the gold standard for diagnosing the behavior of thyroid nodules since the 1980s. More recently, ultrasonography guidance has improved the accuracy of FNAB. Preoperative ultrasonography-guided FNAB has reduced the number of diagnostic surgeries for thyroid nodules that ultimately prove to be benign. However, a recent large multicenter study from the United States showed that up to 26% of FNAB of thyroid nodules were still indeterminate and a median of 34% (range 14%–48%) of patients with indeterminate cytology undergoing surgery had thyroid cancer.[9] Up to a 48% risk of malignancy in indeterminate thyroid nodules is too high to recommend watchful waiting.[1,3,9] In 2007, the United States National Cancer Institute sponsored a conference to review cytologic terminology for thyroid lesions in which experts have proposed the Bethesda classification for reporting thyroid cytopathology.[10] By this classification, the indeterminate thyroid nodules are placed into 3 different categories of cytologic diagnosis: (1) atypia of undetermined significance/follicular lesion of undetermined significance, (2) follicular or oncocytic (Hürthle cell) neoplasm/suspicious for follicular or oncocytic (Hürthle cell) neoplasm, (3) suspicious for malignant cells. Predicted probabilities of cancer in these 3 categories are 5% to 15%, 15% to 30%, and 60% to 75%, respectively.[11] Because FNAB cannot provide a definitive diagnosis for indeterminate thyroid nodules, most of these require a diagnostic thyroid lobectomy. However, only 10% to 40% of such nodules ultimately prove to be malignant. If FNAB could reliably give the preoperative diagnosis of these benign nodules, these unnecessary surgeries with expenses and risks would be avoided. Furthermore, once thyroid lobectomy confirms cancer, completion thyroidectomy is usually offered to the patient as a standard of care to minimize the risk of persistent/recurrent disease and to facilitate radioactive iodine therapy. Optimal treatment of choice for such a patient would be an up-front total thyroidectomy if the diagnosis of thyroid cancer could be established by FNAB beforehand.[1,11]

Cytologic assessment of FNAB remains the best-established diagnostic tool for the evaluation of thyroid nodules, and molecular markers are increasingly being used as adjuncts to cytology to improve diagnosis and to better predict the treatment outcome and prognosis of thyroid lesions.[1,2,11] Several molecular markers, alone and in combination, have been studied in FNAB of thyroid nodules and thyroidectomy specimens.[1–11] This article focuses on the major molecular markers that hold the promise of prognostic value.

PROGNOSTIC APPLICATIONS OF MOLECULAR MARKERS IN THYROID CANCER

Several molecular markers have been associated with the prognosis of thyroid cancer. Even though some markers are promising, BRAF mutation is the best-defined prognostic marker in molecular thyroid medicine.[1]

BRAF Mutation and Prognosis of Thyroid Cancer

The results of a multicenter study suggest that the presence of BRAF mutation predicts a poorer clinical prognosis in papillary thyroid carcinoma because of the strong association of this mutation with high rates of extrathyroidal extension, lymph node metastasis, advanced disease stage, and recurrent/persistent disease.[12] Several subsequent studies have also confirmed these associations.[13–20] BRAF mutation has also been associated with loss of radioiodine avidity of recurrent papillary thyroid carcinoma, which makes the disease refractory to radioiodine treatment.[12,16–18,21–24]

In a 15-year median follow-up study, Elisei and colleagues[25] showed that BRAF mutation correlates with the worst outcome independently from the other clinicopathologic features of the disease. They suggested that these BRAF-positive patients are not only at a higher risk for persistence/recurrence but also for death. A recent international multicenter study also confirmed the strong association of BRAF mutation with mortality of papillary thyroid carcinoma.[24]

Contrary to these reports that BRAF mutation is associated with poor prognosis in papillary thyroid carcinoma, there are studies from Italy, Portugal, and especially from Asia reporting that there is no correlation between the presence of BRAF mutation and high-risk clinicopathologic features, prognosis, or disease-free survival in papillary thyroid carcinoma.[26–30]

Two Korean studies reported very high (up to 79%) prevalence of BRAF mutations in their cohort of a population with papillary thyroid carcinoma. They found no significant association between the presence of BRAF mutation and tumor size, extrathyroidal extension, multifocality of the tumor, or lymph node metastasis. They therefore proposed that BRAF mutation does not serve as a prognostic factor in Korean patients with classic papillary carcinoma or papillary microcarcinoma, and should not independently alter the management.[30,31]

RAS Mutation, RET/PTC Rearrangement, PAX8/PPAR Rearrangement, and Prognosis of Thyroid Cancer

Several studies have reported that RAS mutations are associated with thyroid cancer. However, the prognostic value of RAS mutations remains unclear, because these mutations are not specific for thyroid cancer and can occur with a significant prevalence in benign thyroid nodules.[32–34] RET/PTC rearrangement has been found in classic papillary thyroid carcinoma and has been associated with a high rate of lymph node metastases and lower stage of disease at presentation and is suggested to be a marker of a better prognosis.[2,35] However, more information is required to confirm whether it is a marker of more favorable behavior of thyroid cancer. The isolated detection of PAX8/PPAR rearrangement is neither diagnostic nor prognostic for follicular thyroid carcinoma but may warrant further diagnostic molecular analysis. The correlation of PAX8/PPAR rearrangement and prognosis in patients with follicular thyroid carcinoma is not yet well-defined.[36]

TERT Promoter Mutations and Prognosis of Thyroid Cancer

In 2013, 2 different studies showed that TERT promoter mutations are highly prevalent in advanced/aggressive thyroid cancers, particularly in those harboring BRAF or RAS mutations.[37,38] Therefore, TERT promoter mutations may be biomarkers of tumor progression and used as relevant prognostic markers for patients with thyroid cancer in the near future if further studies can validate these initial reports.

THERAPEUTIC APPLICATIONS OF MOLECULAR MARKERS IN THYROID CANCER

BRAF Mutation in the Management of Thyroid Cancer

Mutations of the BRAF gene are frequently observed in human cancers.[31,39,40] In thyroid tumors, BRAF mutation is restricted to papillary, poorly differentiated, and anaplastic carcinomas.[2,41] BRAF mutation is the most common genetic alteration and has been found in approximately 45% (range 29%–83%) of papillary thyroid carcinomas.[41–54] It is highly prevalent in classic papillary carcinoma and tall cell variant but rare in the follicular variant.[2,12] Detection of this mutation in thyroid FNAB specimens is highly diagnostic for papillary carcinoma.[2,52,55] Therefore, testing for BRAF mutation in thyroid FNAB specimens can establish the diagnosis of papillary thyroid carcinoma in a significant portion of cases with indeterminate or atypical cytology.

There is still debate about whether total thyroidectomy or thyroid lobectomy should be performed for low-risk patients with differentiated thyroid cancer, including papillary microcarcinoma, and whether prophylactic central neck dissection should be chosen in patients with thyroid cancer with no preoperative or intraoperative evidence of metastatic lymph nodes. Because decision making is challenging in these circumstances, molecular testing might be helpful in determining the ideal extent of thyroidectomy and neck dissection in these patients.

BRAF mutation, extrathyroidal extension, and multifocality

Extrathyroidal extension and multifocality contribute to an increased risk of recurrence or persistence of thyroid cancer. Up to 20% of recurrent/persistent thyroid cancers arise in the thyroid remnant.[4,26,56,57] A residual thyroid cancer in the remnant can invade the trachea, esophagus, or nearby neurovascular structures and require aggressive surgical treatment. Yip and colleagues[58] found that BRAF mutation–positive papillary thyroid carcinomas require higher rates of reoperations compared with those without BRAF mutation. Moreover, Howell and colleagues[59] reported a high risk of recurrent papillary thyroid carcinoma in elderly patients (more than 65 years old) with the BRAF mutation. Any recurrent/persistent thyroid cancer may significantly contribute to the morbidity and mortality of the patient. A strong association between BRAF mutation and extrathyroidal extension has been found in patients with thyroid cancer.[4,12,21,58,60] Moreover, Lupi and colleagues[61] found a strong association between BRAF mutation and absence of tumor capsule in papillary thyroid carcinoma. An increased incidence of extrathyroidal extension and multifocality has been reported even in patients with papillary microcarcinoma with the BRAF mutation.[4,57,62,63] Both extrathyroidal extension and multifocality are most often appreciated in the pathologic examination of the thyroidectomy specimen. However, preoperative determination of the BRAF status could be useful to predict the potential risk of extrathyroidal extension and multifocality and this information could possibly help the surgeon and the patient in weighing the risks and benefits of a more extended or aggressive surgery as an initial treatment.

BRAF mutation and lymph node metastasis

Most thyroid cancer recurrences come in the form of lymph node metastases.[4,13,58] The prevalence of lymph node metastasis has been found to be higher in patients with thyroid cancer who harbor the BRAF mutation.[4,12,21,26,27,31,58–60,64–66] Furthermore, the BRAF mutation has been associated with high rates of cervical recurrence and with reoperation.[13,56] Occult metastases of thyroid cancer in the central or even in the lateral compartments of the neck can be missed at the time of initial thyroidectomy and this may contribute to high rates of cervical recurrence and reoperation. Routine preoperative examination of the central and lateral neck by ultrasonography should be done for thyroid nodules suspicious for malignancy by clinical examination and/or cytology, and certainly in BRAF mutation–positive patients with thyroid cancer, in order to decide whether a neck dissection should be added to initial thyroidectomy.[58] Prophylactic central neck dissection could be recommended to all BRAF mutation–positive patients with thyroid cancer if proved to reduce cervical recurrence and reoperation rates in this patient population. Until then, prophylactic central neck dissection cannot be mandated because of the significant risks and morbidity of this surgery in the absence of a clearly defined benefit. However, reoperative central neck dissection has been reported to have an increased risk of complications compared with primary surgery,[67,68] Tufano and colleagues[13] suggested that reoperative central neck dissection can be performed as safely and effectively as primary central neck dissection when treating central compartment nodal metastases but not remnant recurrences. Nevertheless, they noted that there are still risks that should be carefully weighed by the multidisciplinary team and the patient to make the decision on the individual management strategy for each patient.[13]

BRAF mutation and distant metastasis

Distant metastases are not common in differentiated thyroid cancer but, when they occur, they are always adversely associated with prognosis and survival. Kebebew and colleagues[14] reported that BRAF mutation is associated with distant metastasis in patients with only classic papillary thyroid carcinoma. However, according to a recent meta-analysis by Tufano and colleagues,[4] no statistically significant relationship has been found between BRAF mutation and distant metastasis in thyroid cancer.

BRAF mutation, and American Joint Commission for Cancer stage of disease

The American Joint Commission for Cancer staging system for thyroid cancer defines stage III/IV as cases with T3/T4 tumors or any T with lymph node metastasis or distant metastasis in patients more than 45 years old. A statistically significant association between BRAF mutation and advanced stage of thyroid cancer has been reported in several studies.[12,21,25] However, even papillary microcarcinoma can have an aggressive course in the presence of BRAF mutation.[4,57,62,63] The association between BRAF and papillary microcarcinoma and prognosis/behavior needs to be studied further.

RAS Mutation in the Management of Thyroid Cancer

RAS mutations frequently occur in follicular thyroid carcinoma as well as follicular variant of papillary thyroid carcinoma and usually predict low-risk follicular-pattern thyroid cancers. It is the most common mutation found in follicular thyroid carcinoma. However, RAS mutations are not specific for thyroid cancer and they can occur in follicular thyroid adenomas with a significant prevalence.[32,33] Because it is difficult to differentiate follicular lesions from each other in thyroid FNAB samples, diagnostic use of the presence of RAS mutations in thyroid FNAB specimens is controversial.[2,3]

Follicular adenomas with RAS mutations may be the precursors of follicular thyroid carcinoma. Furthermore, the encapsulated follicular variant of papillary thyroid carcinoma is associated with RAS mutation, whereas the infiltrative follicular variant of papillary thyroid carcinoma is associated with BRAF mutation. Therefore, RAS-positive encapsulated follicular variants of papillary thyroid carcinoma have the potential to be treated conservatively, whereas BRAF-positive variants may require more aggressive treatment.[32–34] However, the use of detection of RAS mutation in decision making for the initial treatment (lobectomy vs total thyroidectomy) of thyroid cancers is not yet widely accepted.

RET/PTC and PAX8/PPAR Rearrangement in the Management of Thyroid Cancer

RET/PTC rearrangement is a genetic alteration that is found in approximately 20% of sporadic papillary thyroid carcinomas. It is typically more common in tumors from children, young adults, and those with a history of radiation exposure.[2] Because RET/PTC rearrangement can be detected in thyroid FNAB, it might be a diagnostic marker for papillary thyroid carcinomas. Salvatore and colleagues[52] reported that detection of RET/PTC rearrangement in addition to BRAF mutation refines the diagnosis of papillary thyroid carcinoma and helps with tailoring the initial treatment. RET/PTC rearrangement is associated with a high rate of lymph node metastases and may warrant meticulous examination of central and lateral neck lymph nodes.[35] However, prospective evidence for the utility of detection of RET/PTC rearrangement is still needed in order to consider the implementation of a test for RET/PTC into clinical practice.

PAX8/PPAR rearrangement is the second most common mutation found in follicular thyroid carcinoma. Like RAS, it is typically more common in young patients with follicular thyroid carcinoma. However, it is not specific for follicular thyroid carcinoma, because it has been found in both malignant and benign thyroid neoplasms.[2,3,33] Hence, it remains unclear whether this rearrangement indicates in situ/preinvasive follicular thyroid carcinoma.[36]

Implications of Molecular Markers for Targeted Therapy in the Management of Thyroid Cancer

As understanding of molecular biology has evolved, a few molecules have emerged as promising targets for the treatment of thyroid cancer.[5] In 2 different studies, Carlomagno and colleagues[69,70] showed that RET kinase inhibitors prevent the growth of human PTC cell lines harboring RET/PTC rearrangement. They also showed that sorafenib (a multikinase inhibitor) inhibits the growth of RET/PTC-positive thyroid cancer cells both in vitro and in vivo. Two other clinical trials showed that sorafenib has promising clinical activity with acceptable toxicity in patients with metastatic and radioiodine-refractory thyroid cancer.[71,72] Kim and colleagues[73] showed that another multikinase inhibitor (sunitinib) effectively inhibits signaling from RET/PTC kinase in an experimental model. Sunitinib has also been tested in clinical trials for radioiodine-refractory, unresectable differentiated thyroid cancer.[2] More recently, BRAF kinase inhibitors have been developed and seem to be more potent than sorafenib.[5] Some specific BRAF kinase inhibitors that show their activity preferentially in BRAF mutation–positive tumor cells have shown therapeutic efficacy in vitro.[5,6] Because BRAF is downstream of RET and RAS in the signaling cascade, BRAF inhibitors may be effective in tumors with other mutations that are upstream of BRAF in the cascade.[2] Inhibition of different components of various signaling pathways for thyroid cancer development are still under investigation and various molecular targeted therapy agents are being developed to individualize the treatment of patients with thyroid cancer with specific tumor mutations.

FUTURE TRENDS AND CONCLUSIONS

1. Molecular testing may help decision making when considering the extent of thyroidectomy for cytologically defined cancer and cytologically indeterminate thyroid nodules that are *BRAF* positive.

2. Molecular testing may offer more individualized surgical management based on prognosis.
3. Molecular testing may provide more individualized adjuvant therapy and postoperative follow-up.
4. Molecular testing may provide the basis for the development of novel targeted agents.

REFERENCES

1. Xing M, Haugen BR, Schlumberger M. Progress in molecular-based management of differentiated thyroid cancer. Lancet 2013;381:1058–69.
2. Nikiforova MN, Nikiforov YE. Molecular genetics of thyroid cancer: implications for diagnosis, treatment and prognosis. Expert Rev Mol Diagn 2008;8:83–95.
3. Mehta V, Nikiforov YE, Ferris RL. Use of molecular biomarkers in FNA specimens to personalize treatment for thyroid surgery. Head Neck 2013;35:1499–506.
4. Tufano RP, Teixeira GV, Bishop J, et al. BRAF mutation in papillary thyroid cancer and its value in tailoring initial treatment: a systematic review and meta-analysis. Medicine (Baltimore) 2012;91:274–86.
5. Bozec A, Ilie M, Lassalle S, et al. Usefulness of ancillary methods for diagnosis, prognosis and targeted therapy in thyroid pathology. Curr Med Chem 2013;20: 639–54.
6. Lassalle S, Hofman V, Ilie M, et al. Clinical impact of the detection of BRAF mutations in thyroid pathology: potential usefulness as diagnostic, prognostic and theragnostic applications. Curr Med Chem 2010;17:1839–50.
7. Mitsutake N, Miyagishi M, Mitsutake S, et al. BRAF mediates RET/PTC-induced mitogen-activated protein kinase activation in thyroid cells: functional support for requirement of the RET/PTC-RAS-BRAF pathway in papillary thyroid carcinogenesis. Endocrinology 2006;147:1014–9.
8. Handkiewicz-Junak D, Czarniecka A, Jarzab B. Molecular prognostic markers in papillary and follicular thyroid cancer: current status and future directions. Mol Cell Endocrinol 2010;322:8–28.
9. Wang CC, Friedman L, Kennedy GC, et al. A large multicenter correlation study of thyroid nodule cytopathology and histopathology. Thyroid 2011;21:243–51.
10. Baloch ZW, LiVolsi VA, Asa SL, et al. Diagnostic terminology and morphologic criteria for cytologic diagnosis of thyroid lesions: a synopsis of the National Cancer Institute Thyroid Fine-Needle Aspiration State of the Science Conference. Diagn Cytopathol 2008;36:425–37.
11. Nikiforov YE, Ohori NP, Hodak SP, et al. Impact of mutational testing on the diagnosis and management of patients with cytologically indeterminate thyroid nodules: a prospective analysis of 1056 FNA samples. J Clin Endocrinol Metab 2011;96:3390–7.
12. Xing M, Westra WH, Tufano RP, et al. BRAF mutation predicts a poorer clinical prognosis for papillary thyroid cancer. J Clin Endocrinol Metab 2005;90:6373–9.
13. Tufano RP, Bishop J, Wu G. Reoperative central compartment dissection for patients with recurrent/persistent papillary thyroid cancer: efficacy, safety, and the association of the BRAF mutation. Laryngoscope 2012;122:1634–40.
14. Kebebew E, Weng J, Bauer J, et al. The prevalence and prognostic value of BRAF mutation in thyroid cancer. Ann Surg 2007;246:466–70.
15. Kim TH, Park YJ, Lim JA, et al. The association of the BRAF(V600E) mutation with prognostic factors and poor clinical outcome in papillary thyroid cancer: a meta-analysis. Cancer 2012;118:1764–73.

16. Xing M. BRAF mutation in papillary thyroid cancer: pathogenic role, molecular bases, and clinical implications. Endocr Rev 2007;28:742–62.
17. Xing M. Prognostic utility of BRAF mutation in papillary thyroid cancer. Mol Cell Endocrinol 2010;321:86–93.
18. Nikiforova MN, Nikiforov YE. Molecular diagnostics and predictors in thyroid cancer. Thyroid 2009;19:1351–61.
19. Basolo F, Torregrossa L, Giannini R, et al. Correlation between the BRAF V600E mutation and tumor invasiveness in papillary thyroid carcinomas smaller than 20 millimeters: analysis of 1060 cases. J Clin Endocrinol Metab 2010;95:4197–205.
20. Elisei R, Viola D, Torregrossa L, et al. The BRAF(V600E) mutation is an independent, poor prognostic factor for the outcome of patients with low-risk intrathyroid papillary thyroid carcinoma: single-institution results from a large cohort study. J Clin Endocrinol Metab 2012;97:4390–8.
21. Riesco-Eizaguirre G, Gutierrez-Martinez P, Garcia-Cabezas MA, et al. The oncogene BRAF V600E is associated with a high risk of recurrence and less differentiated papillary thyroid carcinoma due to the impairment of Na+/I- targeting to the membrane. Endocr Relat Cancer 2006;13:257–69.
22. Barollo S, Pennelli G, Vianello F, et al. BRAF in primary and recurrent papillary thyroid cancers: the relationship with (131)I and 2-[(18)F]fluoro-2-deoxy-D-glucose uptake ability. Eur J Endocrinol 2010;163:659–63.
23. Mian C, Barollo S, Pennelli G, et al. Molecular characteristics in papillary thyroid cancers (PTCs) with no 131I uptake. Clin Endocrinol (Oxf) 2008;68:108–16.
24. Xing M, Alzahrani AS, Carson KA, et al. Association between BRAF V600E mutation and mortality in patients with papillary thyroid cancer. JAMA 2013;309:1493–501.
25. Elisei R, Ugolini C, Viola D, et al. BRAF(V600E) mutation and outcome of patients with papillary thyroid carcinoma: a 15-year median follow-up study. J Clin Endocrinol Metab 2008;93:3943–9.
26. Ito Y, Yoshida H, Maruo R, et al. BRAF mutation in papillary thyroid carcinoma in a Japanese population: its lack of correlation with high-risk clinicopathological features and disease-free survival of patients. Endocr J 2009;56:89–97.
27. Fugazzola L, Puxeddu E, Avenia N, et al. Correlation between B-RAFV600E mutation and clinico-pathologic parameters in papillary thyroid carcinoma: data from a multicentric Italian study and review of the literature. Endocr Relat Cancer 2006;13:455–64.
28. Liu RT, Chen YJ, Chou FF, et al. No correlation between BRAFV600E mutation and clinicopathological features of papillary thyroid carcinomas in Taiwan. Clin Endocrinol (Oxf) 2005;63:461–6.
29. Trovisco V, Soares P, Preto A, et al. Type and prevalence of BRAF mutations are closely associated with papillary thyroid carcinoma histotype and patients' age but not with tumour aggressiveness. Virchows Arch 2005;446:589–95.
30. Ahn D, Park JS, Sohn JH, et al. BRAFV600E mutation does not serve as a prognostic factor in Korean patients with papillary thyroid carcinoma. Auris Nasus Larynx 2012;39:198–203.
31. Kim TY, Kim WB, Song JY, et al. The BRAF mutation is not associated with poor prognostic factors in Korean patients with conventional papillary thyroid microcarcinoma. Clin Endocrinol (Oxf) 2005;63:588–93.
32. Gupta N, Dasyam AK, Carty SE, et al. RAS mutations in thyroid FNA specimens are highly predictive of predominantly low-risk follicular-pattern cancers. J Clin Endocrinol Metab 2013;98:E914–22.
33. Witt RL, Ferris RL, Pribitkin EA, et al. Diagnosis and management of differentiated thyroid cancer using molecular biology. Laryngoscope 2013;123:1059–64.

34. Rivera M, Ricarte-Filho J, Knauf J, et al. Molecular genotyping of papillary thyroid carcinoma follicular variant according to its histological subtypes (encapsulated vs. infiltrative) reveals distinct BRAF and RAS mutation patterns. Mod Pathol 2010;23:1191–200.
35. Adeniran AJ, Zhu Z, Gandhi M, et al. Correlation between genetic alterations and microscopic features, clinical manifestations, and prognostic characteristics of thyroid papillary carcinomas. Am J Surg Pathol 2006;30:216–22.
36. Theoharis C, Roman S, Sosa JA. The molecular diagnosis and management of thyroid neoplasms. Curr Opin Oncol 2012;24:35–41.
37. Liu X, Bishop J, Shan Y, et al. Highly prevalent TERT promoter mutations in aggressive thyroid cancers. Endocr Relat Cancer 2013;20:603–10.
38. Landa I, Ganly I, Chan TA, et al. Frequent somatic TERT promoter mutations in thyroid cancer: higher prevalence in advanced forms of the disease. J Clin Endocrinol Metab 2013;98:E1562–6.
39. Xing M. BRAF mutation in thyroid cancer. Endocr Relat Cancer 2005;12: 245–62.
40. Davies H, Bignell GR, Cox C, et al. Mutations of the BRAF gene in human cancer. Nature 2002;417:949–54.
41. Nikiforova MN, Kimura ET, Gandhi M, et al. BRAF mutations in thyroid tumors are restricted to papillary carcinomas and anaplastic or poorly differentiated carcinomas arising from papillary carcinomas. J Clin Endocrinol Metab 2003;88: 5399–404.
42. Fukushima T, Suzuki S, Mashiko M, et al. BRAF mutations in papillary carcinomas of the thyroid. Oncogene 2003;22:6455–7.
43. Fugazzola L, Mannavola D, Cirello V, et al. BRAF mutations in an Italian cohort of thyroid cancers. Clin Endocrinol (Oxf) 2004;61:239–43.
44. Namba H, Nakashima M, Hayashi T, et al. Clinical implication of hot spot BRAF mutation, V599E, in papillary thyroid cancers. J Clin Endocrinol Metab 2003;88: 4393–7.
45. Puxeddu E, Moretti S, Elisei R, et al. BRAF(V599E) mutation is the leading genetic event in adult sporadic papillary thyroid carcinomas. J Clin Endocrinol Metab 2004;89:2414–20.
46. Trovisco V, Vieira de Castro I, Soares P, et al. BRAF mutations are associated with some histological types of papillary thyroid carcinoma. J Pathol 2004; 202:247–51.
47. Xing M, Vasko V, Tallini G, et al. BRAF T1796A transversion mutation in various thyroid neoplasms. J Clin Endocrinol Metab 2004;89:1365–8.
48. Xu X, Quiros RM, Gattuso P, et al. High prevalence of BRAF gene mutation in papillary thyroid carcinomas and thyroid tumor cell lines. Cancer Res 2003; 63:4561–7.
49. Cohen Y, Xing M, Mambo E, et al. BRAF mutation in papillary thyroid carcinoma. J Natl Cancer Inst 2003;95:625–7.
50. Kim KH, Kang DW, Kim SH, et al. Mutations of the BRAF gene in papillary thyroid carcinoma in a Korean population. Yonsei Med J 2004;45:818–21.
51. Kimura ET, Nikiforova MN, Zhu Z, et al. High prevalence of BRAF mutations in thyroid cancer: genetic evidence for constitutive activation of the RET/PTC–RAS–BRAF signaling pathway in papillary thyroid carcinoma. Cancer Res 2003;63:1454–7.
52. Salvatore G, Giannini R, Faviana P, et al. Analysis of BRAF point mutation and RET/PTC rearrangement refines the fine-needle aspiration diagnosis of papillary thyroid carcinoma. J Clin Endocrinol Metab 2004;89:5175–80.

53. Sedliarou I, Saenko V, Lantsov D, et al. The BRAFT1796A transversion is a prevalent mutational event in human thyroid microcarcinoma. Int J Oncol 2004;25: 1729–35.
54. Soares P, Trovisco V, Rocha AS, et al. BRAF mutations and RET/PTC rearrangements are alternative events in the etiopathogenesis of PTC. Oncogene 2003; 22:4578–80.
55. Cohen Y, Rosenbaum E, Clark DP, et al. Mutational analysis of BRAF in fine needle aspiration biopsies of the thyroid: a potential application for the preoperative assessment of thyroid nodules. Clin Cancer Res 2004;10:2761–5.
56. Mazzaferri EL, Jhiang SM. Long-term impact of initial surgical and medical therapy on papillary and follicular thyroid cancer. Am J Med 1994;97:418–28.
57. Niemeier LA, Kuffner Akatsu H, Song C, et al. A combined molecular-pathologic score improves risk stratification of thyroid papillary microcarcinoma. Cancer 2012;118:2069–77.
58. Yip L, Nikiforova MN, Carty SE, et al. Optimizing surgical treatment of papillary thyroid carcinoma associated with BRAF mutation. Surgery 2009;146:1215–23.
59. Howell GM, Carty SE, Armstrong MJ, et al. Both BRAF V600E mutation and older age (≥ 65 years) are associated with recurrent papillary thyroid cancer. Ann Surg Oncol 2011;18:3566–71.
60. Xing M, Clark D, Guan H, et al. BRAF mutation testing of thyroid fine-needle aspiration biopsy specimens for preoperative risk stratification in papillary thyroid cancer. J Clin Oncol 2009;27:2977–82.
61. Lupi C, Giannini R, Ugolini C, et al. Association of BRAF V600E mutation with poor clinicopathological outcomes in 500 consecutive cases of papillary thyroid carcinoma. J Clin Endocrinol Metab 2007;92:4085–90.
62. Lee X, Gao M, Ji Y, et al. Analysis of differential BRAF(V600E) mutational status in high aggressive papillary thyroid microcarcinoma. Ann Surg Oncol 2009;16: 240–5.
63. Lin KL, Wang OC, Zhang XH, et al. The BRAF mutation is predictive of aggressive clinicopathological characteristic in papillary thyroid microcarcinoma. Ann Surg Oncol 2010;17:3294–300.
64. Abubaker J, Jehan Z, Bavi P, et al. Clinicopathological analysis of papillary thyroid cancer with PIK3CA alterations in a Middle Eastern population. J Clin Endocrinol Metab 2008;93:611–8.
65. Musholt TJ, Schönefeld S, Schwarz CH, et al. Impact of pathognomonic genetic alterations on the prognosis of papillary thyroid carcinoma. Langenbecks Arch Surg 2010;395:877–83.
66. Sykorova V, Dvorakova S, Ryska A, et al. BRAFV600E mutation in the pathogenesis of a large series of papillary thyroid carcinoma in Czech Republic. J Endocrinol Invest 2010;33:318–24.
67. White ML, Gauger PG, Doherty GM. Central lymph node dissection in differentiated thyroid cancer. World J Surg 2007;31:895–904.
68. Low TH, Delbridge L, Sidhu S, et al. Lymph node status influences follow-up thyroglobulin levels in papillary thyroid cancer. Ann Surg Oncol 2008;15: 2827–32.
69. Carlomagno F, Vitagliano D, Guida T, et al. Efficient inhibition of RET/papillary thyroid carcinoma oncogenic kinases by 4-amino-5-(4-chloro-phenyl)-7-(t- butyl)pyrazolo[3,4-d]pyrimidine (PP2). J Clin Endocrinol Metab 2003;88: 1897–902.
70. Carlomagno F, Anaganti S, Guida T, et al. BAY 43-9006 inhibition of oncogenic RET mutants. J Natl Cancer Inst 2006;98:326–34.

71. Gupta-Abramson V, Troxel AB, Nellore A, et al. Phase II trial of sorafenib in advanced thyroid cancer. J Clin Oncol 2008;26:4714–9.
72. Kloos RT, Ringel MD, Knopp MV, et al. Phase II trial of sorafenib in metastatic thyroid cancer. J Clin Oncol 2009;27:1675–84.
73. Kim DW, Jo YS, Jung HS, et al. An orally administered multitarget tyrosine kinase inhibitor, SU11248, is a novel potent inhibitor of thyroid oncogenic RET/papillary thyroid cancer kinases. J Clin Endocrinol Metab 2006;91:4070–6.

Decision Making for Diagnosis and Management

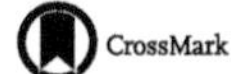

Algorithms from Experts for Molecular Testing

Jeffrey Bumpous, MD[a], Miranda D. Celestre, MD[a], Edmund Pribitkin, MD[b,*], Brendan C. Stack Jr, MD[c]

KEYWORDS

- Thyroid nodule • Thyroid cancer • Ultrasonography
- Fine-needle aspiration cytology • Biomarkers • Molecular classifier

KEY POINTS

- Assessment of risk of thyroid nodules requires understanding of clinical, demographic, imaging, cytopathologic, and now biomarker profiles; none of these factors alone represents a sufficient decision-making factor.
- Ultrasonography represents an accurate and cost-effective imaging modality for evaluating the thyroid, cervical lymphatics, and postoperative thyroid bed.
- Most solid or mixed thyroid nodules greater than 1 cm should undergo cytologic evaluation before surgery with increasing consideration for universal or selective use of biomarker assays.
- Biomarkers such as *Braf* add value to standard cytopathology in identifying suspected well-differentiated thyroid cancers.
- Biomarkers have prognostic value and with additional confirmatory information may help decision making regarding extent of surgical treatment and application of adjuvant treatments.

Disclosures: No disclosures (J. Bumpous); National Institutes of Health grant on PET detector development, PI ECOG/ACRIN 6685, AO Faculty (B.C. Stack); Consultant, Stryker Corporation (E. Pribitkin).

[a] Division of Otolaryngology-Head and Neck Surgery, University of Louisville, Louisville, KY, USA; [b] Department of Otolaryngology-Head and Neck Surgery, Jefferson University College of Medicine, 925 Chestnut Street, 6th Floor, Philadelphia, PA 19107, USA; [c] Department of Otolaryngology-Head and Neck Surgery, University of Arkansas for Medical Sciences, Little Rock, AR, USA

* Corresponding author.

E-mail address: edmund.pribitkin@jefferson.edu

Otolaryngol Clin N Am 47 (2014) 609–623

http://dx.doi.org/10.1016/j.otc.2014.04.007

oto.theclinics.com

INTRODUCTION

In 2013, in the United States, it was estimated that 60,220 new cases of thyroid cancer would be diagnosed and 1850 deaths would be caused by thyroid cancer.[1] Thyroid cancer affects women more often than men and usually occurs in people between the ages of 25 and 65 years.[2] The incidence of this malignancy has been increasing over the last decade.[2] Approximately 60,000 thyroid surgeries are performed annually, of which 33% (20,000) are thyroid lobectomies.[3]

Thyroid cancer risk factors include a history of radiation, goiter, a family history of thyroid disease, the female gender, and the Asian race.[4] Established clinical prognostic factors in well-differentiated thyroid cancer include age greater than 40 years, extrathyroidal/extracapsular invasion, vascular invasion, male gender, follicular disease, and tumors greater than 4 cm. Lymph node status does not seem to affect disease-free survival.

Risk of a nodule being malignant include size, cold nodule status, ultrasonographic (US) features (microcalcifications and increased nodular vascularity), a neck radiation exposure history, a family history in 1 or more first-degree relatives, associated lymphadenopathy on presentation, cytopathology (Bethesda grade) (**Box 1**, **Table 1**), and biomarker results (Afirma [Gene Expression Classifier Veracyte, Inc, San Francisco, CA, USA], MiRInform Thyroid [Asuragen, Inc, Austin, TX, USA], Thyroseq [University of Pittsburgh, Pittsburgh, PA, USA], microRNA).[5,6]

Molecular testing is a developing modality to be used judiciously in clinical practice. Much needs to be studied and reported regarding optimal and cost-effective use of molecular testing in the context of nodular thyroid disease (**Table 2**). This article includes cases that we hope show how molecular biomarker testing of thyroid nodule fine-needle aspirates (FNA) may be appropriately leveraged in a thyroid surgical practice (**Table 3**).

Box 1
The Bethesda system for reporting thyroid cytopathology: recommended diagnostic categories

I. Nondiagnostic or unsatisfactory
- Cyst fluid only
- Virtually acellular specimen
- Other (eg, obscuring blood, clotting artifact)

II. Benign
- Consistent with a benign follicular nodule (includes adenomatoid nodule, colloid nodule)
- Consistent with lymphocytic (Hashimoto) thyroiditis in the proper clinical context
- Consistent with granulomatous (subacute) thyroiditis
- Other

III. Atypia of undetermined significance or follicular lesion of undetermined significance

IV. Follicular neoplasm or suspicious for a follicular neoplasm
- Specify if Hürthle cell (oncocytic) type

V. Suspicious for malignancy
- Suspicious for papillary carcinoma

Suspicious for medullary carcinoma

Suspicious for metastatic carcinoma

Suspicious for lymphoma

Other

VI. Malignant

Papillary thyroid carcinoma

Poorly differentiated carcinoma

Medullary thyroid carcinoma

Undifferentiated (anaplastic) carcinoma

Squamous cell carcinoma

Carcinoma with mixed features (specify)

Metastatic carcinoma

Non-Hodgkin lymphoma

Other

From Baloch ZW, Alexander EK, Gharib H, et al. Overview of diagnostic terminology and reporting. In: Cibas ES, Ali SZ. The Bethesda system for reporting thyroid cytopathology. New York: Springer, 2010; with permission.

Table 1
The Bethesda system for reporting thyroid cytopathology: implied risk of malignancy and recommended clinical management

Diagnostic Category	Risk of Malignancy (%)	Usual Management[a]
Nondiagnostic or unsatisfactory	1–4	Repeat FNA with US guidance
Benign	0–3	Clinical follow-up
Atypia of undetermined significance or follicular lesion of undetermined Significance	~5–15[b]	Repeat FNA
Follicular neoplasm or suspicious for a follicular neoplasm	15–30	Surgical lobectomy
Suspicious for malignancy	60–75	Near-tota1 thyroidectomy or sugica1 lobectomy[c]
Malignant	97–99	Near-total thyroidectomy[c]

Abbreviation: FNA, fine-needle aspiration.

[a] Management may depend on other factors (eg, clinical, sonographic) besides the FNA interpretation.

[b] Estimate extrapolated from histopathologic data from patients with repeated atypicals.

[c] In the case of suspicious for metastatic tumor or a malignant interpretation indicating metastatic tumor rather than a primary thyroid malignancy, surgery may not be indicated.

From Cibas ES, Ali SZ. The Bethesda system for reporting thyroid cytopathology. Am J Clin Pathol 2009;132:658–65; with permission.

Table 2
Analysis of thyroid nodule cytopathology process and optimization

Component	Description	Optimization
Pathology	Follicular-derived lesions and neoplasms have overlapping features Certain neoplasms (eg, classic papillary carcinoma) have characteristic features	Development of tests distinguishing the pathobiological nature of lesions
FNA operator	Aspiration technique Capillary (nonaspiration) technique	Cellular specimen reflecting the architectural pattern of cell proliferation
Specimen processing	Direct smears Liquid-based slides Cell block Collection in molecular preservative	Slides: monolayer of well-preserved and well-stained cells without artifacts Ancillary studies: preservation of nucleic acid and protein molecules
Interpretation and reporting	Bethesda classification (6 tiered)	Standardization and application of criteria for uniform diagnostic practice
Ancillary studies	Molecular markers: BRAF, RAS, RET/PTC, PAX8/PPAR-γ Immunohistochemical markers: HBME-1, galectin-3, CITED-1 Others under development	High sensitivity and specificity for malignant neoplasms

From Ohori NP, Schoedel KE. Thyroid cytology: challenges in the pursuit of low-grade malignancies. Radiol Clin North Am 2011;49:435–51; with permission.

Table 3
Bethesda classification of FNA compared with the usefulness of currently available molecular marker testing

Thyroid Cytology	
Classes of FNA Results	**Usefulness of Molecular Testing**
Negative (II)	Not useful
Rule out follicular neoplasm (III)	Useful
Follicular neoplasm (IV)	Most useful
Suspicious for malignancy (V)	Probably useful (30%–40% still benign at pathology)
Positive (VI)	Not useful

CASES FOR DISCUSSION

Case 1: Incidentally Noted Thyroid Nodule on Carotid Ultrasound

- A 54-year-old man presented with an incidental 1.5-cm mixed cystic solid nodule noted on carotid vascular US. Diagnostic US-guided FNA biopsy (FNAB) was performed. The interpretation was benign colloid goiter, but the case was reviewed by a second pathologist, who made the following comment: "If malignancy is suspected in this solitary thyroid follicular lesion, malignancy cannot be definitively excluded until the questionable mass is completely excised and examined histologically. Clinical correlation is required to determine the next course of action."

Bumpous

The context of this case is a very familiar scenario: a nodule incidentally noted during a diagnostic carotid vascular study. On the US (**Fig. 1**), you can see some of the features that are classic: this nodule meets size criteria (>1 cm), is heterogeneous with cystic and solid features, and merits an FNAB. As you look at the Doppler flow, it is mostly a peripheral pattern, which points toward a benign process; however, the patient underwent an US-guided aspiration biopsy, which showed a follicular aspirate with some blood and colloid. We now get into a situation that I think this case frames nicely. Pathology's statement here is that a malignancy is suspected and it cannot be definitively excluded. By a disclaimer at the bottom of the report, you get the impression that it is benign, but there is no certainty as to

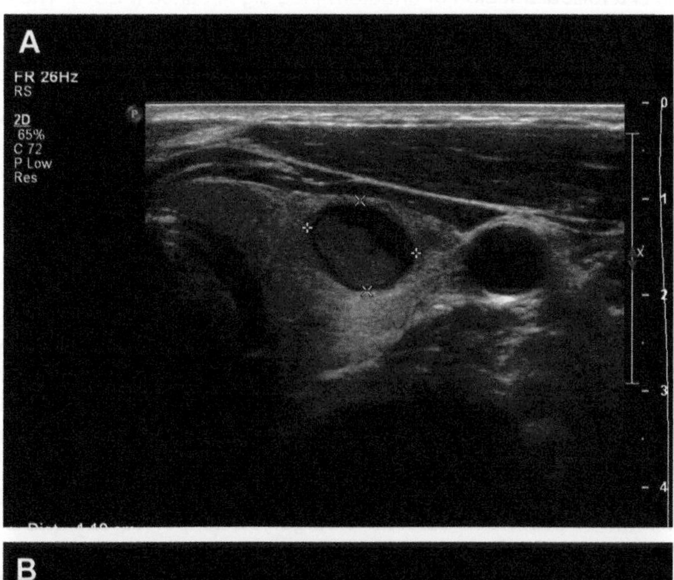

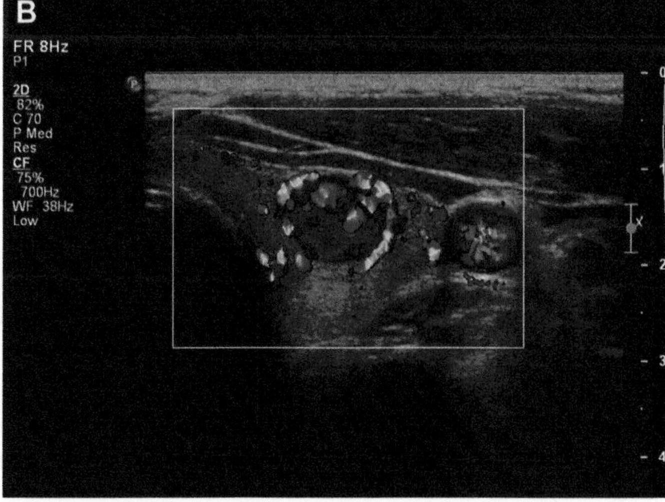

Fig. 1. (*A*) 1.2-cm by 1.0-cm left thyroid lobe lesion, complex cyst, axial view. (*B*) Same lesion as (*A*) in axial view with the Doppler setting on showing peripheral vascularity.

what it is. So, do you proceed with lobectomy, which is the most aggressive approach, or do you repeat the FNA? If you could increase certainty, do you include molecular panels for evaluation of the nodule, or is this a patient who you have a conversation with and simply feel comfortable observing? I think all of these options may have a role depending on the clinical context. If you were doing molecular testing, you would have an informed conversation with the patient and involve the patient in the decision making. What could be the results of the test? How would that influence us? Who pays for the test?

Pribitkin

This is a very common scenario, in which the pathologist does not translate the descriptive diagnosis into the corresponding Bethesda classification category. I would say that this is a follicular lesion of undetermined significance (FLUS). The key here is determining the prevalence of malignancy in your patient population with FLUS on FNAB. At Jefferson, we can tell the patient with this FLUS cytology that about 15% of patients with a similar cytology will have a final diagnosis of cancer. I also tell the patient that almost all these cancers are low grade, slowly increasing in size, not likely to cause death or significant morbidity. In other series of patients featuring a 25% to 40% prevalence of malignancy in FLUS cytologies, it is more reasonable to recommend a thyroid lobectomy. At Jefferson, we would recommend that this patient undergo a repeat US-guided FNAB with molecular panel testing.

Stack

Speaking to the point that Dr Pribitkin made regarding the prevalence of malignancy in your institution, when these diagnoses are made by your pathologist, one might ask, “Well how do you do that?” Random conversations between the surgeon and the pathologist may never arrive at any conclusive data. Our approach at the University of Arkansas for Medical Sciences is to hold a monthly meeting among the surgeons, pathologists, and the radiologists. It is our equivalent of a thyroid cancer tumor board, and we review the pathology of all the cases. Now, some of the pathology will be cytology and will be presented before the surgery. Often, these cases are evaluated retrospectively, so we have the benefit of having cytology and then having operative findings, which include the final pathology. We are able to present these together and engage in conversations that refine our approach to cancer diagnosis. I believe this an important way that you can reach this understanding of the prevalence of malignancy within the various Bethesda classifications of cytology, given the various different interpretations that may come from your pathologists from within your institution.

Bumpous

The tumor board is an outstanding idea. We do the same thing. When you have a high volume, you are able to make those kinds of conclusions. If you do not have a high volume, you have to look at the data throughout your area and look at what leading practices are doing in your area at the university centers. Let us say it is a 15% incidence of a malignancy in FLUS in your center, then I think you can either use the Afirma MiRInform Thyroid, or Thyroseq tests. All have a relatively high negative predictive value at that level of prevalence. When you go up a little higher to a 25% prevalence of malignancy in your FLUS patients, then MiRInform Thyroid demonstrates a diminishing negative predictive value, but both Afirma and Thyroseq hold up in the terms of the negative predictive value. So, in that situation, you would favor doing the Afirma or Thyroseq test as a rule-out negative predictive value test.

Case 2: Asymptomatic Thyroid Mass

- A 50-year-old woman presented with a several-year history of a right thyroid mass. She complained of no symptoms such as dysphagia or airway compromise. The lesion had recently been noticed by a new primary care provider, and referral was made for evaluation and management. On evaluation, the patient had a 2-cm palpable right thyroid mass. The remaining examination was normal. The vocal folds were completely functional on examination. US was performed and showed a 2.6-cm right thyroid lesion, which was heterogeneous without microcalcifications. There were flow patterns around the lesion suggestive of thyroiditis.

Stack

Our concern here is not necessarily of a change in the clinical situation triggering concerns about thyroid lymphoma or anaplastic carcinoma, but this is a long-standing problem, which perhaps has been neglected by the patient or by the primary care doctor. When the patient is evaluated more thoroughly, it reveals a 2-cm lesion in greatest diameter by US, which shows some concern for malignancy. There is also another very common finding of altered vascular flow. Certainly, in middle-aged and older females, vascular flow suggestive of thyroiditis is endemic in North America. We see the cytology both by low power and high power (**Fig. 2**). We have a follicular lesion, and so cytology on its own is not able to distinguish between a follicular carcinoma and a follicular adenoma; perhaps we are just looking at an abundance of follicular cells, and it is not a follicular lesion but just follicular cells. So, there are limits to what cytology can give to us in our operative decision making. This would be another case in which molecular testing could be deployed. In our institution, we have 3 excellent thyroid cytopathologists, and we have not been offering molecular testing to these patients, although it would be appropriate to do so here. Likely, we would repeat the needle biopsy, and if it again showed a predominance of follicular cells and was suggestive of follicular lesion, we would likely proceed to an outpatient diagnostic hemithyroidectomy. Now, if we are going to use surgery as part of making a diagnosis, then the next logical question is when do you use frozen sections? Largely, we do not use frozen sections to make decisions regarding proceeding to total thyroidectomy. Occasionally, if we are concerned with papillary cancer, we do a frozen section on a lymph node, but rarely on the thyroid specimen, unless there are clinical indications of aggressive behavior, such as extrathyroidal extension. Frozen sections do not allow for the comprehensive evaluation of a follicular lesion to determine if there are areas where there is vascular or capsular invasion.

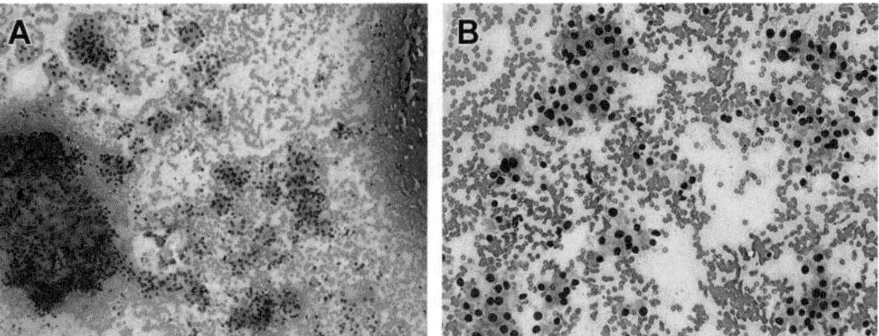

Fig. 2. (*A*) FNA of a follicular at low power. (*B*) FNA of a follicular at high power. (Papanicoloau stain, A&B).

Bumpous
This is another common scenario, in which you have to exercise some cautions; in particular, I think that the image guidance of the biopsy by an experienced ultrasonographer is critical. If you have a situation where you are suspicious of thyroiditis and a follicular process, you are much more likely to obtain follicular features, and those might be coexistent with the other disease. In frozen section, standardizations of processes are very important; in particular, the number of sections taken through a lesion. Simply bivalving the nodule in hopes of determining that this is a follicular carcinoma versus follicular adenoma is unlikely to be a sufficient examination to make that determination. Studies have been quite good at looking at frozen sections, and if you increase the number of sections that are actually done with the nodule, the security of developing that diagnosis is much better. So, there are competencies and processes within pathology which are critical to make frozen section valuable. In my institution, I use frozen sections on a selective basis usually to confirm a clinical suspicion. If I see, for example, fibrous changes or if I am suspicious of muscle invasion, or if I see a lymph node that appears suspicious, that is the context that I clinically consider frozen sections as a support for increasing the extent of surgery.

Pribitkin
I would agree that you need to have the processes in place. I think it is an interesting question in terms of your frozen section. We looked at this many years ago before the era of molecular testing, and what we found was that intraoperative cytology, a touch prep, of the lesion during the procedure was most effective in terms of making a diagnosis. I would urge you to speak with your pathologist to make sure that cytology is done. When we looked at the cost-effectiveness of intraoperative frozen section, we also discovered the reduction in costs arose not from the identification of follicular carcinomas, but rather from the identification of follicular variants of papillary thyroid cancer (FVPTC). At that time, these intraoperative FVPTC diagnoses prompted us to do a total thyroidectomy and saved the patient another operation, therefore making intraoperative cytology cost effective. Interestingly, the FNAB data including preoperative testing with molecular diagnosis show that BRAF and NRAS testing limits the cost-effectiveness of intraoperative cytology. Essentially, you obviate frozen sections by incorporating molecular testing results into your preoperative decision making.

Case 3: Rapidly Enlarging Thyroid Mass

- A 30-year-old man presented with left thyroid mass that had been rapidly growing over 3 months. He self-referred because he was distressed about the possibility of cancer. Physical examination was a healthy young man with a 3-cm left thyroid mass, which was tender to palpation. US and FNA were performed, and 2 lesions were noted. The 3-cm lesion was cystic; its cytology is shown in **Fig. 3**A. There was an adjacent 7-mm left lobe lesion, which was solid and hypervascular; its cytology is shown in **Fig. 3**B.

Stack
Unlike our previous case, this is a new finding clinically and, therefore, raises the concern on the part of the patient and the providers as to whether there is cancer. A patient may come in with 1 clinical finding, and others are found on US. The actual lesion that prompted presentation had benign cytology with a very classic appearance where the colloid has this bubble gum pink/purple appearance spread across the slide

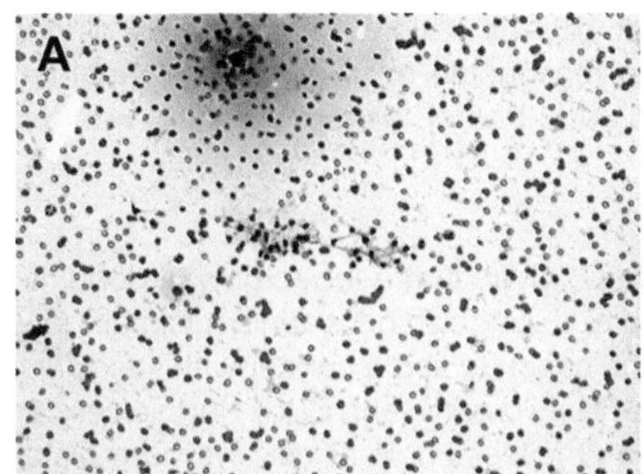

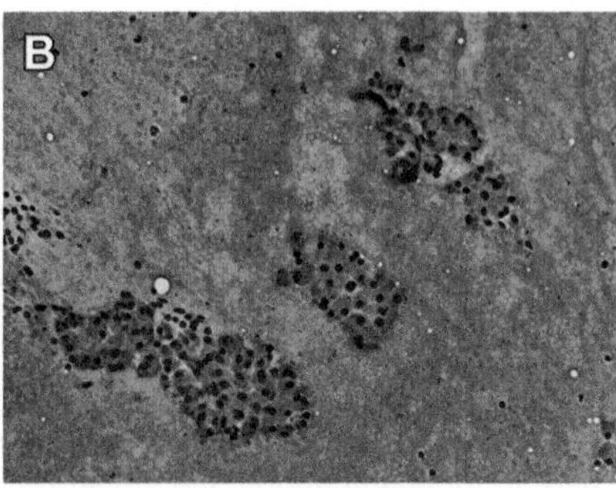

Fig. 3. (*A*) Bubble gum colloid appearance of a benign colloid nodule aspirate. (*B*) FNA of a Hürthle cell lesion. (Papanicoloau stain, A&B).

(see **Fig. 3**A). The incidentally found lesion adjacent to the dominant lesion is concerning for a Hürthle cell neoplasm. Again, we have a similar quandary: what options would we offer for the patient? Is this a patient for whom molecular testing would be appropriate? And would you base your surgical decisions on intraoperative frozen sections? So I am very interested to hear what my colleagues are going to say about this, because this is very similar to our previous case with regards to whether we should offer observation or lobectomy with or without frozen section.

Pribitkin

Seven-millimeter lesions are relatively small, and this is an incidental finding, because, if you were not biopsying the big lesion, you would not have biopsied the 7-mm lesion, unless it had some suspicious characteristics on US. I think you can reassure the patient to some extent by offering molecular testing. The molecular testing would help us to decide whether or not a lobectomy should be done. Given the small size of the lesion, a lobectomy should be sufficient, unless the final pathology revealed an unusual malignancy.

Stack

I appreciate the remarks of Dr Pribitkin, and let me just plays devil's advocate here. You have a lesion that by definition could be a carcinoma. If it was a carcinoma, and you could offer him a thyroidectomy, which would be both a diagnostic and therapeutic given a totally clean contralateral lobe, Dr Bumpous, would this change your approach? Would you forgo perhaps molecular analysis since the final common pathway seems to be coming together? Would you not bother with frozen sections in this particular case but just defer to permanent pathology?

Bumpous

This is a scenario where you have an intersection of science and medicine, and it underscores the importance of informed conversations with your patients. The likelihood of this being malignant is fairly low and, even if it were malignancy, the implications of it are relatively small. On the other hand, if it were an 80-year-old patient, you would feel much more comfortable proceeding perhaps with a more conservative approach. I do not think it is unreasonable to perform a lobectomy on this patient. What you have to inform the patient of in this situation is if there could be findings that might indicate that this was more aggressive. If you have multifocal carcinoma that is found at the time of permanent pathology, maybe this is someone who may have to consider a completion of thyroidectomy. I think that is unlikely given the fact that you have pretty good US examination. You have to provide the patient with the options of repeat FNA or initial FNA with molecular testing. I still think it is reasonable to perform the lobectomy. I agree with Dr Pribitkin's comments earlier, and I do not think proceeding with total thyroidectomy is the first step.

Pribitkin

One of the things to look for on final pathology, given that a lobectomy is done, is a Hürthle cell or follicular malignancy. We have to distinguish between a minimally invasive cancer, where there is just invasion of the capsule, and a cancer with vascular or lymphatic invasion. In the former case, a lobectomy is sufficient. But a Hürthle cell cancer that has vascular invasion, even if it is a small lesion, is at risk for more distant spread. In those situations, we would recommend a total thyroidectomy, so that we can more easily screen for distant metastases with serum thyroglobulin and better follow the patient long-term.

Stack

I appreciate Dr Pribitkin's remarks as far as the surgery is concerned, and in the event that this came back Hürthle cell carcinoma with signs of vascular invasion, I totally concur with completion of total thyroidectomy. My question for Dr Pribitkin is that, given that we know the size of this lesion, and that we have no other surprise findings on final pathology on the left lobe, would he consider doing a left central neck dissection (CND), because of the findings of vascular invasion.

Pribitkin

No, we would not. There are no signs of lymph node enlargement on US or on other types of imaging, and Hürthle cell carcinomas are more likely to spread hematogenously. We would not, therefore, do a CND, especially, given the increased morbidity of a CND performed in conjunction with a completion thyroidectomy 1 to 2 weeks following the initial surgery. If the thyroglobulin remained elevated postoperatively, we would obtain both an iodine radionuclide and a positron emission tomography computed tomography scan to evaluate the patient for distant metastases.

Case 4: Incidentally Discovered Thyroid Mass During Carotid Artery Evaluation

- A 60-year-old man presented with a left thyroid mass incidentally discovered on a vascular duplex study for carotid artery evaluation. His physical examination was normal, and the lesion was not palpable to your examination. A US examination showed a 1.4-cm left thyroid lesion in a background of thyroiditis. There was some increased perilesional vascular flow, and a few microcalcifications were appreciated. An FNA was performed and returned as in **Fig. 4**. In counseling the patient, what advice do you give? He asked if there was a role for molecular testing and you said no. Why?

Stack

Another challenge is when older patients come in with incidental findings, whether it is through PET scanning for surveillance of another cancer or, in this case, a carotid scan. There is some concern about carotid artery disease, and when performing this examination, US reveals a 1.4-cm left thyroid lesion with some concerning findings: there appears to be some increase of vascular flow around the lesion, which is a soft concerning sign that the lesion is malignant. The FNA is performed appropriately, and it returns findings which are classic for papillary thyroid cancer (PTC). What advice would you give to the patient? And given that there appears to be some certainty in the diagnosis, do we need to do molecular testing in this case?

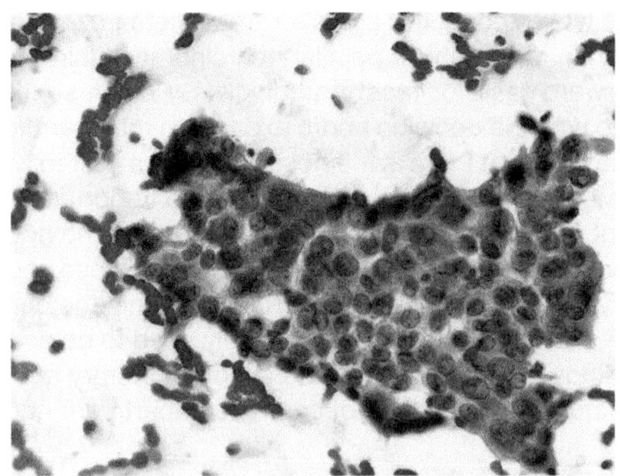

Fig. 4. FNA positive for papillary thyroid cancer. (Papanicoloau stain).

Bumpous

When you have a fairly clear situation, molecular testing does not offer a considerable amount of added value, and it does add cost. There is also some trepidation that I have, as we have a case here that looks very classic: nuclear grooves, papillary type of pathology that is diagnostic for carcinoma. If you had testing that was counter to the diagnosis of papillary carcinoma, would that persuade you from doing at least a lobectomy on this patient, given these cytologic findings? I think in this situation, molecular testing is redundant and could confuse the clinical decision making.

Pribitkin

I agree that this patient requires a total thyroidectomy. If you have confidence in your cytopathology, then there really is no need for intraoperative frozen section. I do not think that you can be faulted, if you do have some concerns about the cytopathology, to get an intraoperative frozen section to increase your level of confidence. Occasionally, there are scenarios where you operate on 1 side of the thyroid and you run into difficulties. If you run into difficulties on 1 side, then, before you go to the other side, get frozen section pathology to confirm the diagnosis, and you may avoid doing a total thyroidectomy in an otherwise very difficult situation. Given that this is a small cancer in an elderly gentleman and the question arises, in what situations would you perform a CND?

Stack

This patient is a clinically N0 neck based on the information that we are given here. With a thyroid gland in situ in the neck, it is difficult to do a comprehensive US evaluation of level 6 to know that there is adenopathy. You have 1 further chance, and that is during the removal of the thyroid, you may find some clinical adenopathy, and again, we are not given that information on this particular case. But finally, we have the American Thyroid Association (ATA) guidelines that we can look to for advice. The ATA guidelines do not recommend routine (prophylactic) CND for T1 and T2 lesions, which would be the category that this lesion falls into. So, absent finding nodes while doing the thyroidectomy, I would not go ahead and do a CND.

Bumpous

I agree wholeheartedly with Dr Stack. I would not routinely perform a CND in this situation. There are some findings that would upstage the patient, such as intraoperative findings of capsular invasion or clinically positive lymphadenopathy. When you have an intermediate-size lymph node, it is again an area where frozen section can assist in your decision, because identifying a papillary carcinoma within the lymph node is a relatively straightforward task for most pathologists. Frozen section analysis of the lymph node can help with the decision about expanding the operation. I always inform the patient preoperatively that there is the possibility that a limited lymph node dissection may be required. I think another issue that is also important is the extent of the central compartment neck dissection. Do you remove all of the nodes that are lateral to the recurrent nerve or can you restrict your dissection to those nodes that are medial to the recurrent nerve? What are the node groupings within the central compartment that need to be assessed, or do all of them routinely need to be assessed? We would be remiss not to acknowledge that the incidence of temporary and permanent hypoparathyroidism is increased in the face of central compartment nodal dissection.

Case 5: Thyroid Mass Post Removal of Parathyroid Adenoma

- A 50-year-old female patient who had had removal of left inferior parathyroid adenoma 1 year previously presented with US showing a right 1-cm thyroid mass with microcalcifications. There was no lymphadenopathy or contralateral thyroid nodules. There was no history of neck irradiation or family history of thyroid cancer. The patient was euthyroid, and the hyperparathyroidism was cured with unilateral exploration. The FNA was suspicious for PTC; BRAF and NRAS were negative (**Fig. 5**A, B).
- The patient underwent right thyroid lobectomy. No lymph nodes were encountered at surgery. Both parathyroids were preserved. Final pathology showed

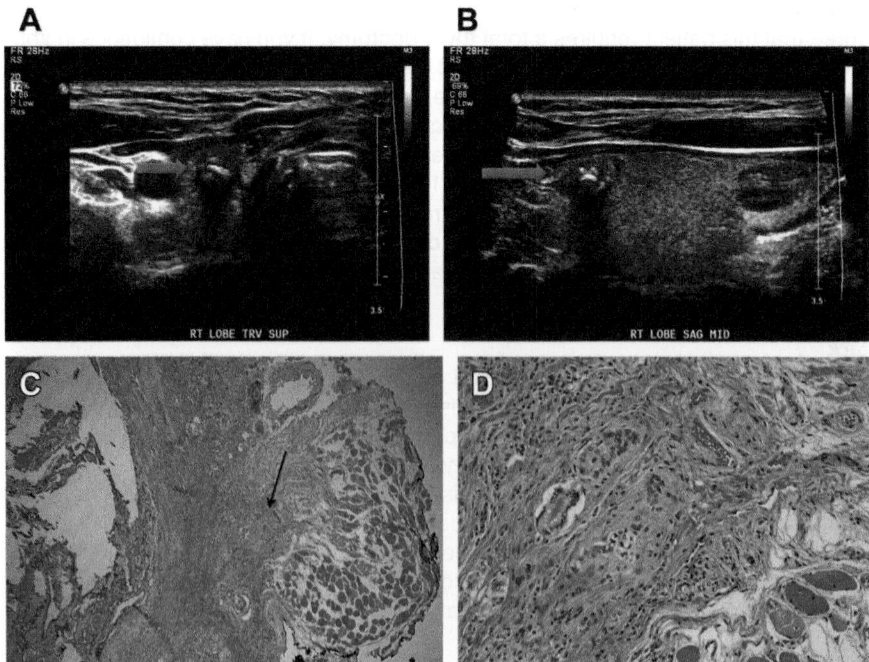

Fig. 5. (*A*) Right thyroid lesion in transverse (axial) view. (*B*) Same lesion as (*A*) in a sagittal view. (*C*) Low-power hematoxylin-eosin view of same lesion as (*A*), *Arrow* area is magnified in *D*. (*D*) High-power hematoxylin-eosin view of same lesion as (*A*), PTC.

8-mm PTC, with 1 focus of extrathyroidal extension of PTC. There were no parathyroids in the specimen (see **Fig. 5**C, D).

Stack

It is important that when you see characteristics that are suspicious on US, it raises your suspicion for doing FNA and ultimately recommending surgery, even if the aspiration is equivocal. Microcalcifications as well as irregular borders on US are worrisome findings. These findings move you up that level to be concerned for a malignancy. Again, no lymphadenopathy was seen on US. When we look at both the longitudinal and the transverse view, we can also get an appreciation of whether the lesion is taller than it is wide, which is also associated with an increasing likelihood of malignancy. The FNA was suspicious for papillary thyroid carcinoma and there was molecular testing done. The molecular testing showed both BRAF and NRAS negative. So the more common molecular tests for malignancy were negative but the cytopathology was suspicious for PTC. Here, we have a lesion that is suspicious but not conclusive papillary thyroid carcinoma. So, what would the recommendation be in terms of initial surgery?

Bumpous

This situation is one in which you have disparate data and you have US findings and cytopathologic findings that are highly suspicious for malignancy, yet your molecular testing is not pointing in that direction. There are a variety of reasons that this can occur. I think that this is a situation in which you exercise caution and have a conversation with the patient: we have features that are pointing to malignancy but not a definitive diagnosis of malignancy, so in my estimation, this is a perfect case for a thyroid lobectomy. With an assessment of either frozen section or permanent section, you have high rates of confidence and good quality control. With frozen section, you may or may not be able to make intraoperative decision making, based on previously discussed parameters.

Stack

In my particular setting, given this lesion has about 60% chance of being PTC. I would start with a thyroid lobectomy. I may or may not, based on the clinical situation, do a frozen, but I would in all likelihood proceed to doing total thyroidectomy at this operative setting. Given the aggressive final pathology, if only a thyroid lobectomy were performed, I would proceed with a completion thyroidectomy. When I do completion thyroid surgery, I assume that there are no functioning parathyroids on the previously operative side, whether it is myself or another surgeon who referred the case. And the fact that the patient had at least 1 parathyroid removed previously does not dissuade me from this more aggressive thyroidectomy posture.

Pribitkin

The 1 bit of data that exists in some of the larger studies, but has not been conclusively proven, is that BRAF-negative low-risk microcarcinomas cases exhibit a far lower mortality and disease recurrence. There is a suggestion that a lobectomy could potentially suffice in these patients, especially if there is concern about a higher risk of having a problem on the other side during the surgery. This patient did undergo just the right thyroid lobectomy, there were no lymph nodes encountered in surgery, everything went very smoothly, and the final pathology showed a microcarcinoma (8 mm), but it did show extrathyroidal extension. The question now is whether one proceeds with a completion thyroidectomy for this microcarcinoma with a little bit of extrathyroidal extension? Is a central neck indicated as well?

Bumpous

The extrathyroidal extension is a finding you should not ignore. I would proceed with a completion thyroidectomy and at least an ipsilateral CND on the side of the lesion. The rationale for doing this is that there is a high rate of a lymph node metastasis, so a CND provides further pathologic staging that would inform decisions regarding adjuvant therapy.

Stack

There are 3 reasons why we want to do a total thyroidectomy: number 1 is that these lesions can be multifocal, and multifocality is both a prognostic and a therapeutic issue in treating thyroid cancer. There is also the issue that remaining thyroid tissue will be an impediment to radioactive iodine, and finally, the use of serum thyroglobulin is not effective, unless a total thyroidectomy has been performed. These are 3 reasons in my mind, in addition to guideline reasons, in addition to the diagnosis of cancer, that we would do completion thyroidectomy. I would concur with the need to do unilateral CND, because now we know that with final pathology, this is at least a T3 lesion with minimal extrathyroidal spread, and it would be a T4 with more extensive extrathyroidal spread.

Case 6: Incidentally Discovered 2.5 cm Nodule

- A 33-year-old patient presents with an incidentally found right 2.5-cm nodule (**Fig. 6**A). There was no lymphadenopathy or contralateral thyroid nodule. There was no history of neck irradiation or a family history thyroid cancer. The patient was euthyroid. FNA showed a follicular neoplasm; BRAF was negative but NRAS positive.

Pribitkin

This is a scenario in which the suspicion for a malignant follicular neoplasm is much higher, and I would offer the patient lobectomy, with possibly a confirmatory frozen section (see **Fig. 6**B). I think one of the issues here is the value of the upfront molecular testing. When we get an NRAS-positive result, there have been some centers that have suggested that this carries an 87% incidence of a malignancy of some type. The most common malignancy is a follicular variant of PTC. Some centers would proceed with a total thyroidectomy, because at the University of Pittsburgh, those individuals who had a follicular variant of papillary cancer also had an additional 50% risk of having a contralateral follicular variant of papillary cancer, even in the presence of a normal lobe on US.

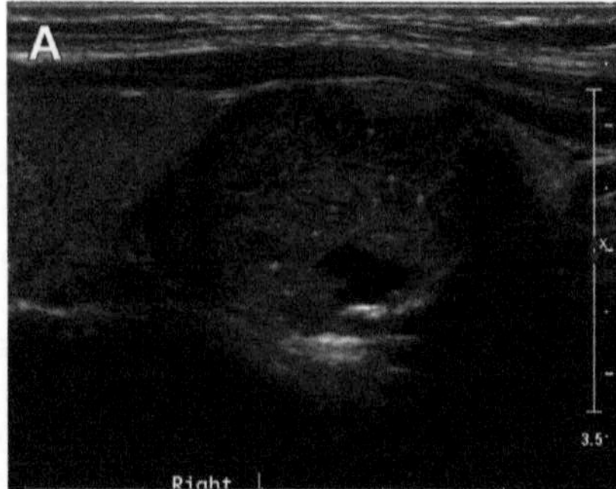

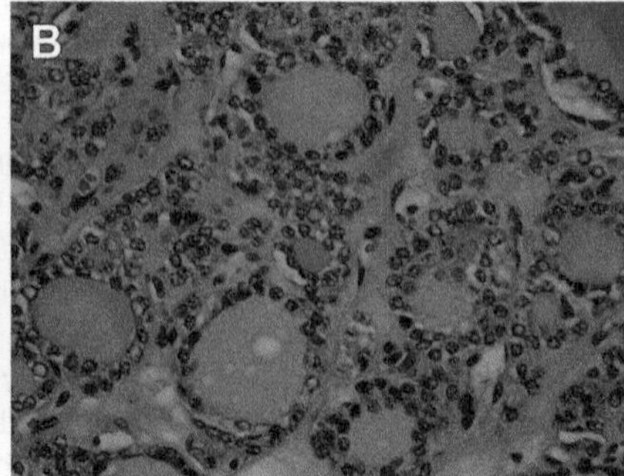

Fig. 6. (*A*) A 2.5-cm right thyroid nodule. (*B*) High-power view of same lesion as (*A*), follicular neoplasm. (hematoxylin-eosin).

Stack

In my practice, we would not be using the molecular testing with any regularity. We would not have that information. We already have the cytology, which raises our index of suspicion that we may be dealing with a malignancy. In this particular situation, I would do a frozen section. Intraoperative frozen sections can help to identify papillary cancer. And based on that information, I would proceed to do a total thyroidectomy, I would do an intraoperative examination of level 6 and do any lymph node dissection that would be indicated based on my intraoperative findings.

REFERENCES

1. American Cancer Society. Cancer facts and figures 2013. Atlanta (GA): American Cancer Society; 2013.
2. Tennvall J, Biörklund A, Möller T, et al. Is the EORTC prognostic index of thyroid cancer valid in differentiated thyroid carcinoma? Retrospective multivariate analysis of differentiated thyroid carcinoma with long follow-up. Cancer 1986;57(7): 1405–14.
3. Vashishta R, Mahalingam-Dhingra A, Lander L, et al. Thyroidectomy outcomes: a national perspective. Otolaryngol Head Neck Surg 2012;147(6):1027–34.
4. Iribarren C, Haselkorn T, Tekawa IS, et al. Cohort study of thyroid cancer in a San Francisco Bay area population. Int J Cancer 2001;93(5):745–50.
5. Nikiforova MN, Wald AI, Roy S, et al. Targeted next-generation sequencing panel (ThyroSeq) for detection of mutations in thyroid cancer. J Clin Endocrinol Metab 2013;98(11):E1852–60. http://dx.doi.org/10.1210/jc.2013-2292.
6. Gupta N, Dasyam AK, Carty SE, et al. RAS mutations in thyroid FNA specimens are highly predictive of predominantly low-risk follicular-pattern cancers. J Clin Endocrinol Metab 2013;98(5):E914–22. http://dx.doi.org/10.1210/jc.2012-3396.

REFERENCES

Index

Note: Page numbers of article titles are in **boldface** type.

Otolaryngol Clin N Am 47 (2014) 625–630
http://dx.doi.org/10.1016/S0030-6665(14)00076-0 oto.theclinics.com
0030-6665/14/$ – see front matter

R

S

T

Moving?

Make sure your subscription moves with you!

To notify us of your new address, find your **Clinics Account Number** (located on your mailing label above your name), and contact customer service at:

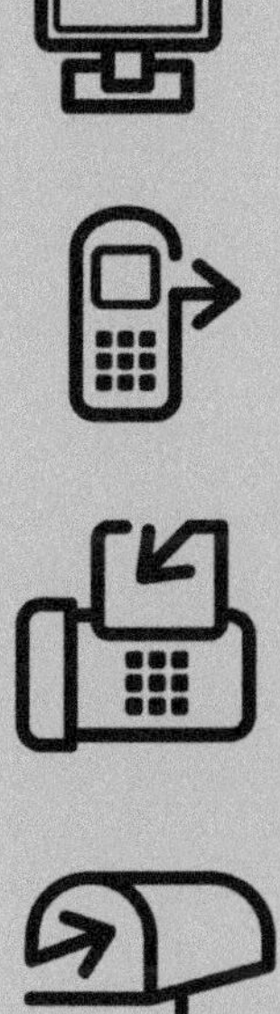

Email: journalscustomerservice-usa@elsevier.com

800-654-2452 (subscribers in the U.S. & Canada)
314-447-8871 (subscribers outside of the U.S. & Canada)

Fax number: 314-447-8029

Elsevier Health Sciences Division
Subscription Customer Service
3251 Riverport Lane
Maryland Heights, MO 63043

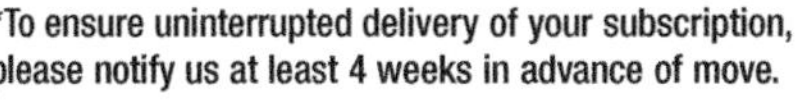

*To ensure uninterrupted delivery of your subscription, please notify us at least 4 weeks in advance of move.

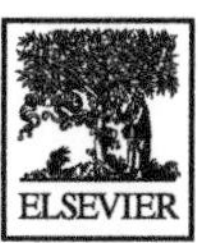

Printed and bound by CPI Group (UK) Ltd, Croydon, CR0 4YY
03/10/2024
01040491-0018